I0095810

# Hardwired but Human, Redefining Strength, Resilience, and Self-Mastery for Men Who Don't Do Therapy

A Field Guide For Men Who Value Grit Over Grief-Talk,

Logic Over Labels But Still Want Peace Of Mind, Purpose,

And Power

Nicci Brochard
&
Dr. Ben Chuba

# Hardwired but Human, Redefining Strength, Resilience, and Self-Mastery for Men Who Don't Do Therapy

A Field Guide For Men Who Value Grit Over Grief-Talk,

Logic Over Labels But Still Want Peace Of Mind, Purpose,

And Power

Copyright©2025

All rights reserved by Nicci Brochard & Dr. Ben Chuba

Published in the United States by Cross Border Publishers.

No part of this publication may be reproduced, stored, or transmitted in any form or by any means electronic, mechanical, photocopying, recording, or otherwise without prior written permission from the author or publisher, except for brief excerpts used in reviews or educational purposes as permitted by law.

This book is protected under U.S. and international copyright laws. Unauthorized reproduction, distribution, or adaptation of any portion of this work may result in legal consequences.

For permissions, licensing, or inquiries, please contact

info@crossborderpublishers.com: www.crossborderpublishers.com

Book Formatting by: Monisha

Book cover design by: *Billy Design*

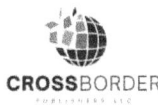

**CROSS**BORDER

New York, London, Quebec

# Contents

## Chapter 5: The Self-Reliant Toolbox — Building a Mental Fitness Routine ............................................................. 36

## Chapter 6: Stoic, Not Stone — Redefining Emotional Resilience ............................................................. 45

## Chapter 7: Anger, Burnout, and the Silent Pressure Cooker ........ 53

## Chapter 8: Relationships Without the Drama or Therapy Talk ... 62

# Introduction

Vulnerability is often equated with weakness; many men have been conditioned to bottle up their emotions, suppress their struggles, and power through life's challenges with sheer will. Yet, beneath the surface, the pressure to maintain this façade of unbreakable toughness can take a toll on mental health, relationships, and personal well-being. Enter *Hardwired but Human: Redefining Strength, Resilience, and Self-Mastery for Men Who Don't Do Therapy*. This book is for the men who value grit over grief-talk, logic over labels, and practicality over emotional self-analysis but still desire to find peace of mind, purpose, and power in their lives.

The premise of this guide is simple: Men have been told for generations that real strength lies in silence, in keeping your head down, and in not sharing your vulnerabilities with others. But what if strength and resilience aren't about avoiding emotions or pushing through pain at all costs? What if they could be about learning to navigate life's struggles in a way that honors both your inherent toughness and your humanity? *Hardwired but Human* challenges the conventional wisdom that men must choose between being stoic and being whole. It offers a new path, one that embraces the complexities of masculinity while providing actionable tools to achieve self-mastery.

This book acknowledges that many men don't want to sit in a therapist's office or engage in endless discussions about feelings. Instead, they want to know how to stay strong and grounded without sacrificing their mental health or happiness. They want real solutions, not labels. They want practical advice, not theoretical frameworks. *Hardwired but Human* offers precisely that—a field guide designed for men who appreciate clarity, logic, and action, all while learning how to balance their inner strength with self-compassion.

Throughout this book, you will explore concepts such as resilience, emotional control, and self-awareness, but these aren't the fluffy, feel-good ideas often peddled in mainstream discussions of mental health. Rather, you'll gain tools that align with the way you already think and operate, presented in a no-nonsense, pragmatic manner. It's not about abandoning your inherent drive for success, your commitment to personal strength, or your need for control. It's about refining those qualities and directing them towards a life that's balanced, fulfilled, and sustainable.

This guide emphasizes the importance of reclaiming your power by taking ownership of your emotional and mental landscape. Far too often, men are told to keep it together at all costs, even if it means suppressing their true feelings. But self-mastery doesn't come from denying or ignoring the emotional currents beneath the surface—it comes from understanding them, managing them, and using them to fuel your drive for greatness, while also fostering the peace and calm necessary to navigate life's inevitable storms.

By the end of *Hardwired but Human*, you will have a deeper understanding of what it means to truly be strong and resilient in today's world. You'll learn that true strength isn't just about physical prowess or the ability to endure—it's about having the emotional intelligence to navigate life's challenges without losing yourself along the way. You'll discover how to develop a mental toolkit that sharpens your decision-making, fortifies your emotional endurance, and builds a sense of inner peace that allows you to stay grounded, no matter what life throws your way.

If you're a man who's ready to redefine what it means to be strong, to embrace resilience on your own terms, and to find the peace of mind, purpose, and power you deserve, this book is for you. *Hardwired but Human* will provide you with the tools, strategies, and insights you need to be a man who not only thrives under pressure but does so with wisdom, clarity, and authenticity. It's time to stop battling your emotions and start mastering them.

Ben and I (Nicci) thank you immensely for choosing our book. We promise you will find in it what you are looking for.

# Chapter 1

## The Tough Shell Myth — Why Strong Men Still Struggle

**Introduction:**

For generations, men have been taught to wear an invisible armor—a tough shell that shields them from the world's harshest blows. The cultural script surrounding masculinity has long demanded that men embody an unwavering resolve, a stoic determination that keeps emotions buried beneath layers of unspoken expectations. But in the real world, where pressure, pain, and struggles are a constant part of life, this armor has become a double-edged sword. While it might seem to protect, it often ends up trapping men in a silent battle, one that chips away at their well-being without them even realizing it.

This chapter delves into the powerful cultural narrative that promotes emotional toughness as a measure of masculinity. We'll explore why the societal expectation for men to "tough it out" has resulted in what I call the "Tough Shell Myth," and how this myth leads to the silent epidemic of high-functioning emotional distress. Men are conditioned to believe that acknowledging their struggles makes them weak, but this mindset only perpetuates the internal turmoil. We'll examine the difference between merely "sucking it up" and the more empowered act of stepping up to face life's challenges—emotionally, mentally, and practically.

# The Cultural Script Around Masculinity and Mental Toughness

The cultural narrative around masculinity is as old as civilization itself. From the warriors of ancient tribes to the rugged, self-reliant heroes of the American frontier, men have been celebrated for their stoicism, physical strength, and emotional fortitude. The ideal man was often portrayed as someone who could endure any hardship, who could suppress his emotions and never falter in the face of adversity. This image of masculinity was not only encouraged but revered, creating a standard for men to live up to that was rooted in silence, endurance, and emotional suppression.

However, this script is deeply flawed. It teaches men that their worth is tied to their ability to be "tough" in every situation—be it physical, emotional, or psychological. The societal pressure to conform to this ideal becomes overwhelming when the expectation is to appear strong at all costs, even when things aren't going well internally. Men are told to "man up," to "get over it," and to keep their heads down and their feelings in check. They are often warned against being "too emotional" or "too soft," as if these qualities were antithetical to masculinity itself.

The idea of mental toughness has been distorted. True mental strength isn't about suppressing emotions or pretending that everything is fine when it clearly isn't. Rather, mental toughness is about having the courage to face one's emotions head-on, to understand their significance, and to use that emotional awareness as a tool for growth. When men embrace emotional suppression, they are denying themselves the chance to be fully human. They become prisoners of a myth—a myth that suggests real men don't feel, and that expressing vulnerability is somehow a sign of weakness.

## The Silent Epidemic of High-Functioning Emotional Distress

While society's demand for emotional restraint may seem benign at first glance, the consequences are far-reaching. Men have internalized this script so deeply that the emotional strain it places on them often goes unnoticed—both by themselves and by those around them. This leads to what I refer to as the silent epidemic of high-functioning emotional distress.

High-functioning emotional distress is a condition where men outwardly appear to be managing well—continuing to go to work, take care of their families, and maintain their responsibilities—while internally, they are struggling to cope with feelings of anxiety, depression, frustration, or isolation. These men often don't seek help, not because they don't need it, but because they don't know how to ask for it without feeling like they're failing to meet the expectations placed upon them.

This silent epidemic is pervasive. Studies show that men are less likely to seek professional help for mental health issues compared to women, in part because they fear being labeled as weak or incapable. The result is that many men live with untreated emotional pain for years, often masking their distress with distractions like work, exercise, or substance use. They may seem to be thriving in the eyes of others, but inwardly, they are fighting a battle that no one knows about.

The fact that these men are functioning at a high level despite their emotional distress speaks to their resilience, but it also underscores the danger of this myth. The more a man buys into the idea that he should be able to handle everything on his own without help, the more likely he is to experience long-term mental and physical health issues. Over time, the strain of maintaining the tough exterior can erode a man's mental clarity, emotional stability, and sense of peace.

The myth that men must be strong at all times creates a toxic environment where men feel like they are constantly failing if they aren't always in control. It's a recipe for burnout, stress, and chronic dissatisfaction. But acknowledging struggle and seeking help doesn't make a man weak—it makes him wise.

## Why Acknowledging Struggle Isn't Weakness—It's Strategic

One of the most important lessons a man can learn is that acknowledging his struggles isn't a sign of weakness. In fact, it's a strategic move toward long-term strength and success. The ability to recognize when you are struggling, and to take steps to address it, is the hallmark of true emotional and mental resilience.

Men who struggle but refuse to acknowledge it often find themselves caught in a cycle of denial, self-criticism, and isolation. They become convinced that their struggles are something to hide, and that admitting them would tarnish their reputation as "strong" men. This fear of vulnerability prevents them from seeking the help or support they need, ultimately causing their struggles to grow unchecked. Over time, the cost of this denial becomes more apparent—whether it's a breakdown in relationships, physical health issues, or emotional burnout.

On the other hand, men who are able to recognize and face their struggles head-on, without shame, are far better equipped to navigate life's challenges. By embracing their vulnerabilities, they gain greater emotional intelligence, which enables them to respond to adversity in a healthier and more strategic manner. Acknowledging one's struggles allows men to take the necessary steps to improve their mental health, seek support, and make adjustments to their lives when necessary. This proactive approach is not a sign of weakness but rather a demonstration of self-awareness and wisdom.

Strength isn't about enduring pain in silence—it's about being capable of facing discomfort and uncertainty with clarity, confidence, and a willingness to seek solutions. In this sense, acknowledging struggle is a strategic move that empowers men to take control of their mental, emotional, and physical well-being.

## The Difference Between "Sucking It Up" and Stepping Up

There's a significant difference between "sucking it up" and stepping up to the challenges that life presents. The phrase "suck it up" has long been used as a shorthand for enduring hardship without complaint, but in reality, it often leads to a dangerous pattern of repression. When men "suck it up," they are merely suppressing their feelings, avoiding their emotional needs, and pretending that everything is fine when it clearly isn't. This approach may appear to work in the short term, but it creates long-term consequences—emotional numbness, relational distance, and burnout.

In contrast, stepping up means facing the challenges head-on and taking responsibility for one's well-being. Stepping up involves acknowledging the difficulty of the situation, understanding the emotions involved, and taking deliberate action to address them. It's not about avoiding or denying pain but about embracing the opportunity to grow through it. Stepping up requires a man to not only confront his emotions but also use them as a source of insight and motivation.

Stepping up is about cultivating resilience, not by ignoring vulnerability but by embracing it as part of the human experience. It's about doing the difficult work of processing emotions, seeking help when necessary, and taking strategic steps toward healing and growth. Unlike the superficial act of "sucking it up," stepping up is an active, empowered choice to take control of your emotional and mental life.

## Conclusion:

The Tough Shell Myth has perpetuated the idea that men must be tough at all costs, that they must suppress their emotions, avoid vulnerability, and keep pushing through life's challenges without ever admitting weakness. This myth has led to a silent epidemic of high-functioning emotional distress among men, who often struggle in isolation because they fear being perceived as weak or incapable. But acknowledging struggle is not a sign of weakness—it's a strategic move toward greater strength, resilience, and emotional intelligence.

Men who are able to step up and confront their struggles head-on, without shame or fear of judgment, are better equipped to navigate the complexities of life. The key to true strength lies not in denying emotions or enduring hardships in silence but in embracing vulnerability as a powerful tool for personal growth. When men learn to step up—by facing their struggles, seeking help when needed, and taking proactive steps toward healing—they can unlock a level of strength that transcends the hollow toughness perpetuated by societal expectations. In doing so, they can finally break free from the constraints of the Tough Shell Myth and embrace a more balanced, empowered version of masculinity.

# Chapter 2

# You're Not Broken — You're Wired for Survival

## Introduction:

From an early age, many men are taught that emotions are something to be conquered—something to ignore or suppress. This idea is rooted in a deep misunderstanding of both biology and psychology. Men, by and large, aren't broken or defective in their emotional responses; instead, they are hardwired for survival. The way men think, react, and behave has been shaped over millennia by evolutionary forces designed to ensure their survival. The challenge, however, is that these evolutionary instincts—rooted in the ancient, primal brain—often clash with modern society's expectations and the emotional complexity of today's world.

In this chapter, we will explore the male brain and behavior through an evolutionary lens, examining how survival instincts shaped the way men think and feel. We will look at the neurological responses that trigger fight, flight, freeze, and even fix reactions, and how these innate responses influence the way men approach the world. We will also discuss how men have been conditioned to react rather than reflect, and why this automatic response often leads to emotional disconnection. Finally, we'll delve into the idea that emotions are not the enemy, but rather valuable data that can provide insights into our behavior and decision-making.

## The Male Brain and Behavior: An Evolutionary Perspective

Human beings, both male and female, are a product of evolution—a biological process shaped by millions of years of natural selection. Our brains, particularly the ones responsible for emotions and survival, have evolved in response to the challenges our ancestors faced. Understanding the evolutionary backdrop of male behavior begins with acknowledging that men, just like women, are driven by biological instincts designed to maximize survival, reproduction, and success in an ever-changing environment.

From an evolutionary standpoint, the male brain is optimized for certain tasks: rapid decision-making, spatial awareness, and physical exertion, to name a few. These traits have long been associated with the "hunter" archetype in early human societies, where men were often tasked with protecting their groups, hunting for food, and confronting threats head-on. Survival depended on quick, decisive action—often in situations that were life-threatening. Because of this, the male brain is wired to respond with high levels of focus and rapid reaction when faced with danger or uncertainty.

This biological wiring has a direct impact on men's emotional and behavioral responses. The brain, particularly the amygdala and the prefrontal cortex, controls emotional reactions, but the amygdala—the brain's "fear center"—is dominant when it comes to survival instincts. It processes threats almost instantaneously, triggering the fight, flight, or freeze responses before the rational part of the brain has a chance to weigh in.

In ancient times, these quick responses were critical. When faced with a saber-toothed tiger or an invading tribe, there was no time for reflection. A decision had to be made immediately: fight for survival, flee to safety, or freeze to avoid detection. These instincts were essential for keeping men alive.

However, in the modern world, these instincts are less adaptive. While the need to react quickly to physical threats has decreased, the emotional and psychological triggers that activate the fight-or-flight response are still present. For example, the stress of a difficult conversation at work, the pressure of financial insecurity, or the emotional strain of a relationship conflict can trigger the same primal reactions as the sight of a predator. The difference is that modern challenges are not typically life-or-death situations, yet the brain still responds as if they are.

## Fight, Flight, Freeze... or Fix?

The well-known "fight or flight" response is only part of the story when it comes to understanding male behavior. In recent years, psychologists and neuroscientists have added a third element to this list: freeze. This response is less commonly discussed but is just as critical to understanding the way men—especially in high-stress situations—deal with emotional or physical threats.

- **Fight**: The fight response is about taking action, engaging in the problem head-on, and overcoming the threat. This reaction is often linked with aggression, anger, or confrontation. The body is flooded with adrenaline, which prepares the individual to either physically defend themselves or stand their ground.

- **Flight**: The flight response is all about escaping the situation, avoiding confrontation, or retreating to safety. This reaction is typically tied to feelings of fear, anxiety, or helplessness. The body prepares to run or avoid the threat, and emotions such as panic and fear often accompany this response.

- **Freeze**: The freeze response occurs when the body becomes immobilized in the face of a threat. This reaction is often linked to feelings of overwhelm, confusion, or helplessness. In extreme situations, the body may temporarily shut down, rendering the individual unable to act or make decisions.

- **Fix**: While not originally part of the fight-or-flight framework, the "fix" response is a critical reaction in understanding modern male behavior. This is when men, rather than fighting, fleeing, or freezing, attempt to immediately solve the problem or "fix" the situation. The idea of fixing problems is deeply embedded in male socialization. Men are often encouraged to be solution-oriented, to find answers and solve challenges quickly, which can be a positive trait. However, this response can also become a double-edged sword. In emotional or relational contexts, men often feel compelled to "fix" the issue without taking the time to understand or process their emotions. In relationships, for example, men might try to resolve a partner's emotional distress without first acknowledging the emotional undercurrent beneath the issue.

The fixation on "fixing" can lead to frustration, miscommunication, and emotional neglect if the underlying feelings aren't addressed. It's essential for men to learn when to step back and listen rather than immediately attempting to solve the problem, as this can ultimately lead to greater emotional health and deeper connections with others.

## How Men Are Conditioned to React, Not Reflect

From a young age, boys are often conditioned to react quickly and decisively, particularly in stressful situations. "Be a man," they're told, "don't cry," and "don't show weakness." These messages, whether explicit or implicit, reinforce the idea that men should act before they feel. This conditioning is rooted in societal and cultural norms that have historically placed value on action over reflection, decisiveness over hesitation, and strength over vulnerability.

This conditioning creates a cycle where men are more likely to react emotionally—either by lashing out in anger, retreating in fear, or becoming numb through inaction—rather than take the time to pause, reflect, and process their emotions. Over time, this lack of reflection leads to emotional suppression, confusion, and disconnect. Men who are taught to react first and reflect later may never take the time to understand the deeper emotional triggers behind their actions. This is where many men go wrong, as they ignore the emotional signals their bodies are giving them in favor of a knee-jerk reaction that doesn't necessarily serve them in the long term.

In today's world, where emotional intelligence and awareness are highly valued, this pattern of reactionary behavior can be counterproductive. It prevents men from being fully present in their relationships, whether with partners, friends, or colleagues. Moreover, it hampers their ability to engage with their own emotional landscape, denying them the opportunity to grow and understand their true feelings.

The good news is that this behavior can be shifted. By learning to embrace reflection over reaction, men can begin to understand the deeper reasons behind their feelings and make decisions that are not solely driven by survival instincts but by thoughtful consideration of the consequences. This shift doesn't require abandoning the survival instincts that are hardwired into the male brain; rather, it's about learning to balance them with the ability to pause, reflect, and choose a response that aligns with their values and goals.

## Emotions Aren't the Enemy—They're Data

One of the most damaging myths surrounding masculinity is the idea that emotions are something to be avoided or overcome. In reality, emotions are not the enemy. They are incredibly valuable data points that provide insight into our inner world. Emotions are our body's way of communicating important information about our environment, our needs, and our desires. They are not inherently good or bad; they are simply signals that we must learn to interpret and respond to.

For example, feelings of anger can provide insight into underlying frustrations or unmet needs. Sadness may indicate a loss or an unmet emotional desire. Fear, while uncomfortable, is a signal that we are facing potential danger or uncertainty. Rather than attempting to suppress or ignore these emotions, men can learn to use them as valuable information to guide their decisions and actions.

Emotions are not a sign of weakness or something to be feared. Instead, they are tools that help men navigate the complexities of life. The key is not to allow emotions to control you, but to allow them to inform your decision-making process. By learning to recognize and understand your emotions, you can respond to them in a way that aligns with your goals and values, rather than simply reacting from a place of fear, anger, or confusion.

## Conclusion:

The male brain is not broken—it is wired for survival. From an evolutionary perspective, men are hardwired to react quickly to threats, often in the form of fight, flight, freeze, or fix. These instincts served our ancestors well in a world where survival depended on immediate action. However, in today's world, these same instincts often lead to emotional disconnection, miscommunication, and an inability to reflect on one's emotions.

Men have been conditioned to react first and reflect later, which can prevent them from fully understanding their emotional landscape. However, by shifting from reactionary behavior to reflective thinking, men can tap into the valuable emotional data that emotions provide.

Learning to embrace emotions as data, rather than an enemy, is the first step toward emotional mastery and deeper self-awareness.

As men, we are not broken, but rather wired for survival. The challenge now is to adapt these hardwired instincts to the complexities of modern life, where reflection, emotional intelligence, and balanced decision-making are as critical to success as raw physical strength and instinctive reaction. When men learn to reflect before reacting, they unlock the ability to navigate life's challenges with clarity, purpose, and authenticity.

# Chapter 3

# Emotions 101 — Read 'Em Without Losing Your Edge

## Introduction:

Emotions are often seen as inconvenient interruptions to logic and action, especially for men conditioned to prioritize grit, discipline, and the absence of vulnerability. Yet, in reality, emotions are not the enemy; they are a part of the intricate fabric of the human experience. Whether they manifest as anger, fear, shame, or pride, emotions provide essential data about our internal states and external environments. The problem arises not when emotions exist but when we fail to understand, identify, and manage them effectively.

For men, who are often discouraged from embracing emotional awareness, this can become a significant hurdle. When emotions are bottled up or ignored, they can manifest in unproductive ways— sabotaging relationships, hindering career progression, and damaging physical and mental health. This chapter offers a practical guide to understanding, identifying, and navigating core emotions, ensuring that they enhance, rather than diminish, your power and effectiveness in life.

We will explore how emotions like anger, shame, fear, pride, and others influence behavior, often unconsciously, and how you can decode these emotions before they hijack your actions. You will learn to identify emotions you may not even realize you're experiencing and how to prevent unspoken emotions from sabotaging your relationships, career, and health. Finally, we'll introduce the "dashboard light" method for emotional awareness, which will provide you with the tools to become more attuned to your emotions while maintaining your edge.

## Practical Guide to Identifying Core Emotions: Anger, Shame, Fear, Pride, and More

One of the first steps in mastering your emotions is being able to identify and name them. Often, we experience a flood of emotions without ever truly understanding what we're feeling. It can be easy to label a complex mix of emotions as "stress" or "frustration" when in fact there are multiple layers at play. By learning to identify core emotions, you gain the power to dissect them and decide how to respond rather than react impulsively.

1. **Anger**: Anger is one of the most commonly misunderstood emotions, especially in men. It's often viewed as aggressive or uncontrollable, yet anger itself is simply a response to perceived injustice, frustration, or threat. It's a natural emotional reaction to situations where we feel powerless, disrespected, or threatened. The key to managing anger lies in distinguishing between the emotion itself and how we choose to express it. When anger arises, it's crucial to pause and assess what triggered it. Is it a real threat, or is it a reaction to a perceived slight? Understanding the root cause of your anger can help you redirect

it productively, instead of letting it cloud your judgment or harm your relationships.

2.  **Shame**: Shame is a powerful and often debilitating emotion that can be particularly challenging for men. It arises when we feel we have failed or fallen short of our own or society's expectations. Shame can lead to feelings of worthlessness or inadequacy and often causes people to hide their true selves. For men, shame is often linked to notions of masculinity—fears of being seen as weak, vulnerable, or ineffective. The first step in addressing shame is recognizing that it's an emotion designed to push us to act according to our values and social norms. However, it becomes toxic when it turns inward and drives us to believe we are fundamentally flawed. Learning to separate the emotion of shame from your sense of self-worth is key to overcoming it.

3.  **Fear**: Fear is a survival mechanism that has kept humanity alive for thousands of years. It's a signal that something important is at stake. Whether it's physical safety or emotional security, fear alerts us to potential danger. However, in modern life, fear is often triggered by perceived threats that are not life-or-death situations—like the fear of failure, rejection, or uncertainty. While fear can be paralyzing, it can also be empowering when harnessed. By acknowledging fear and assessing the level of risk involved, you can decide whether to confront it or let it pass. The key is to prevent fear from hijacking your decision-making

process and instead use it as a guide to help you take calculated action.

4. **Pride**: Pride is often considered a positive emotion, reflecting a sense of accomplishment or self-worth. It's the emotion that drives us to perform at our best and take pride in our work, relationships, and achievements. However, pride can become toxic when it turns into arrogance, leading to overconfidence or a refusal to acknowledge mistakes. The key to healthy pride is humility—recognizing your strengths while also being open to learning and growth. Healthy pride allows you to feel good about your achievements without letting it define your identity or alienate others.

5. **Guilt**: Guilt arises when we believe we've done something wrong or failed to live up to our values. It's closely tied to the desire to make amends and correct mistakes. Guilt can be constructive if it prompts positive change or corrective action. However, when guilt becomes excessive or irrational, it can lead to self-criticism and paralysis. It's important to assess whether your guilt is proportional to the situation and whether it's motivating you to take action or simply holding you in a state of regret.

6. **Sadness**: Sadness is often misunderstood as an inherently negative emotion, but it serves an essential purpose. It's a response to loss, disappointment, or unmet expectations. Sadness signals that something important is missing or that a change is needed. While it's a painful emotion, sadness allows us to process

grief and loss, ultimately helping us heal. Men may struggle with sadness because it's often associated with vulnerability, but learning to experience sadness without shame can open the door to emotional depth and empathy.

## What Most Men Feel but Can't Name—and How to Decode It

There are many emotions that men experience but often can't name. These emotions don't always fit neatly into categories like anger, sadness, or pride, and as a result, they get muddled or overlooked. Common examples include:

- **Frustration**: Frustration occurs when we feel blocked from achieving our goals or desires. It can manifest as a general sense of irritation or an acute feeling of being stuck. While frustration can be a motivator for change, it often gets bottled up or directed outward toward others when it's not processed properly.

- **Anxiety**: Anxiety is often a blend of fear and worry about potential future events. Men may not always recognize their anxiety for what it is, mistaking it for stress or pressure. However, anxiety can become overwhelming if not acknowledged and dealt with.

- **Loneliness**: Men, particularly those who are conditioned to be self-reliant, may experience loneliness but struggle to articulate it. This feeling can arise from social isolation, emotional disconnection, or the inability to meet their deeper emotional needs. The silent suffering of loneliness can have serious implications for mental health and relationships if not addressed.

- **Envy**: Envy is a common emotion that stems from the desire for what others have. Men may not always recognize envy, as it is often masked by competitiveness or a desire to achieve more. However, unchecked envy can lead to unhealthy comparisons and dissatisfaction with one's own life.

By learning to decode these emotions, you can become more attuned to what's happening beneath the surface. This awareness gives you the power to address these feelings directly and make more intentional choices about how to respond.

## How Unspoken Emotions Sabotage Relationships, Careers, and Health

When emotions go unspoken or unacknowledged, they have the potential to sabotage key aspects of life, including relationships, careers, and overall health. Emotions, when repressed, create tension within and can affect one's interactions with others, often leading to conflict, misunderstandings, and a lack of fulfillment.

- **Relationships**: In relationships, unspoken emotions such as frustration, anger, or fear can fester over time. Men often suppress these emotions to avoid appearing weak or vulnerable. However, this can lead to emotional distance and a breakdown in communication. When emotions are not communicated openly, partners may feel neglected or misunderstood. Over time, this lack of emotional transparency erodes trust and intimacy, potentially leading to relationship breakdowns.

- **Careers**: In the workplace, emotions like fear of failure or anxiety can affect job performance and decision-making. When men suppress these feelings, they may struggle with burnout, stress, or poor judgment. Additionally, emotions like pride and frustration can manifest as overconfidence or defensiveness, creating tension with colleagues or superiors. Emotional awareness allows men to navigate workplace dynamics more effectively, enabling better collaboration, leadership, and personal growth.

- **Health**: Chronic suppression of emotions can lead to physical and mental health issues, such as high blood pressure, digestive problems, anxiety, or depression. When emotions are ignored or repressed, the body responds with stress, which can take a significant toll on overall health. Recognizing and addressing emotions early on helps to prevent long-term health complications and promotes overall well-being.

## The "Dashboard Light" Method for Emotional Awareness

One of the most effective ways to stay attuned to your emotions without losing your edge is by using the "dashboard light" method of emotional awareness. Just as the dashboard lights in a car indicate when something needs attention—whether it's low fuel, engine trouble, or a warning about tire pressure—emotions act as signals that something requires your attention.

Here's how the dashboard light method works:

1. **Identify the Emotion**: When you feel something intense— anger, fear, shame, pride—take a moment to pause and identify it. Ask yourself, "What am I feeling right now?" Try to pinpoint the emotion without judgment. Recognizing that you're experiencing an emotion is the first step in taking control.

2. **Assess the Situation**: Once you've identified the emotion, assess the situation that triggered it. What caused this emotional response? Is it a situation where action is required, or is it simply an emotional signal asking you to pause and reflect?

3. **Decide on the Response**: After identifying and understanding the emotion, decide how to respond. If the emotion requires action (like anger or frustration), use it as a motivator to make constructive changes. If the emotion is something like sadness or fear, consider how you can process it in a healthy way—perhaps by talking to someone, journaling, or taking time to reflect.

4. **Monitor and Adjust**: Just as a car's dashboard lights don't stay on indefinitely (they signal, and then you address the issue), emotions don't need to dominate your state of mind. Check in with yourself regularly to see if any new emotional signals are present, and take action as needed to address them.

By using the dashboard light method, you can stay emotionally aware without letting your emotions take control of your behavior or decision-making. This method allows you to process your emotions in real-time, enhancing emotional intelligence and maintaining your focus and edge.

## Conclusion:

Emotions are not the enemy—they are valuable data that can guide us toward better decision-making, deeper relationships, and improved well-being. Understanding and identifying core emotions like anger, fear, shame, pride, and others can give you greater control over your actions and reactions. By learning to decode what you're truly feeling, you can prevent unspoken emotions from sabotaging your relationships, career, and health. The "dashboard light" method offers a practical framework for becoming more emotionally aware, enabling you to process emotions effectively without losing your edge.

As men, it's time to embrace emotional intelligence not as a weakness but as a tool for greater strength and self-mastery. By understanding the emotional signals that arise within you and learning to respond strategically, you unlock the power to navigate life's challenges with clarity, purpose, and emotional resilience.

# Chapter 4

# The Control Illusion — What You Can (and Should) Actually Master

**Introduction:**

In a world that constantly shifts—filled with uncertainty, chaos, and unpredictable events—control can feel like the ultimate answer. We strive to control our circumstances, our outcomes, our environments, and, sometimes, even the people around us. The desire for control is often tied to our need for security and certainty, yet this yearning for control can lead us down a destructive path. It is an illusion—the idea that we can control everything, or even most things, in our lives.

In this chapter, we will challenge the myth of absolute control and reframe our understanding of what we truly have the power to master. True control isn't about dominating situations or forcing outcomes; it's about mastering ourselves. It's about controlling our reactions, our routines, and our responses to external stimuli. This internal mastery is where true power lies—when we learn to navigate life with emotional intelligence and strategic action.

We will also explore the concept of power versus force, a key distinction that separates those who act with true internal strength from those who rely on external dominance. And finally, we'll dive into tactical tools—breathing, reframing, and body regulation—that can help you maintain control over your reactions and emotional responses, especially in high-stress moments.

## Reframing Control: Not Over Others, But Over Reactions, Routines, and Responses

The first step in mastering control is understanding where control truly lies. In many aspects of life, control is a fleeting illusion. We can try to control the actions of others, the direction of our career, or the outcomes of specific projects, but ultimately, there are many factors outside of our influence. External forces, from the actions of others to the fluctuations of the market, are beyond our control. When we attempt to control these elements, we often find ourselves frustrated, stressed, and disillusioned.

However, there is one area of life where control is not only possible but essential: the control of our own reactions, routines, and responses. This form of internal control is empowering because it doesn't rely on external validation or circumstances. It rests solely on our ability to govern ourselves.

- **Reactions**: Our reactions are often automatic, shaped by our past experiences, emotional triggers, and ingrained behaviors. Learning to control our reactions means taking responsibility for how we respond to situations. This might sound simple, but it is one of the hardest things to master. In high-pressure moments, our immediate reactions are often driven by fear, anger, or frustration, which can cloud our judgment. However, by learning to pause before reacting, we can choose how we respond—

whether with calmness, clarity, or even silence. The ability to control your reactions is one of the greatest tools for emotional and mental strength.

- **Routines**: Routines are the backbone of success, discipline, and stability. A well-established routine brings structure to an otherwise chaotic world. When we have control over our routines—whether in the morning, at work, or before bed—we create a sense of order in our lives. Routines allow us to conserve mental energy, reduce decision fatigue, and maintain focus on what matters most. When we control our routines, we can prioritize the activities that promote growth, well-being, and productivity. The key is to recognize that routines are not about rigid perfection; they are about consistency and intentionality.

- **Responses**: Our responses are our conscious choices in any given situation. Unlike reactions, which are often automatic, responses require awareness and deliberation. For example, if we are confronted with criticism or conflict, our immediate reaction might be defensiveness. However, our response is a conscious decision about how to handle that moment—whether by engaging with empathy, asserting ourselves calmly, or taking a step back to evaluate the situation. Mastering our responses gives us the power to act with intention and integrity, regardless of the external circumstances.

When we focus on what we can control—our reactions, routines, and responses—we liberate ourselves from the frustration that comes with trying to control things outside of our power. We recognize that we can't control everything, but we can always control how we show up in the world.

## Power vs. Force: Choosing Internal Strength Over External Dominance

In many parts of our lives, we are taught to equate power with dominance—being able to assert control over others, influence outcomes, or bend the world to our will. But this is a limited, and ultimately unfulfilling, view of power. There is a distinction between power and force that, when understood, can dramatically shift the way we approach challenges and relationships.

- **Power** is the ability to influence and navigate situations through internal strength, wisdom, and emotional intelligence. It is rooted in self-mastery, empathy, and confidence. People who operate with power are in control of their emotions, their behavior, and their interactions. They don't need to force outcomes because their energy naturally attracts respect and cooperation. Power is quiet but commanding; it doesn't seek to dominate but to align.

- **Force**, on the other hand, is the attempt to control or dominate others through aggression, manipulation, or coercion. It is an external exertion of will that relies on pushing, forcing, or overpowering situations to get what one wants. While force can lead to short-term gains or successes, it often comes at the cost of relationships, trust, and long-term fulfillment. Force is reactive; power is proactive. Force requires external validation, while power is self-sustaining.

Choosing internal power over external force is a shift in mindset that leads to greater emotional resilience and personal success. When we choose power, we are choosing to act from a place of inner strength. We trust that our actions, when aligned with our values, will lead to the outcomes we desire. We don't need to force things to happen because we have faith in our own abilities and decisions.

In relationships, careers, and life, power allows us to influence others without exerting control over them. We can guide, inspire, and lead by example, rather than by force. In this way, power is a sustainable, long-term approach to success, while force is a temporary fix that can burn bridges and drain energy.

## Tactical Tools: Breathing, Reframing, and Body Regulation in High-Stress Moments

Mastering control over ourselves is not only about mindset; it's also about having practical tools at our disposal to manage high-stress moments. When we are under pressure, our ability to react quickly and appropriately can be compromised by emotions like anger, anxiety, or panic. To maintain control in these moments, we need techniques that help us regain our emotional and mental equilibrium. Below are three key tactical tools: breathing, reframing, and body regulation.

1. **Breathing**: Breath is often the most overlooked but most powerful tool for managing stress. When we are stressed,

anxious, or overwhelmed, our breathing becomes shallow and rapid, which can exacerbate the feeling of panic. By consciously slowing down our breath, we can activate the parasympathetic nervous system (our "rest and digest" system), which calms the body and mind. The act of deep breathing shifts our focus from the stressor to the breath itself, grounding us in the present moment.

A simple but effective breathing technique is the 4-7-8 method:

- Inhale through your nose for a count of 4.

- Hold your breath for a count of 7.

- Exhale slowly through your mouth for a count of 8.

This technique helps to reduce anxiety, calm the nervous system, and restore clarity. By incorporating deep breathing into your routine, you can use it as a tool to manage high-stress situations and regain control when emotions run high.

2. **Reframing**: Reframing is the ability to change the way we perceive a situation. When faced with a challenge or stressful event, our initial reaction may be to view it as a threat or an obstacle. However, reframing allows us to see the same situation from a different perspective, often one that is more empowering and solution-focused.

For example, if you're facing a difficult conversation with a colleague or partner, you might initially feel defensive or anxious. Reframing that situation might involve seeing it as an opportunity for growth, connection, and understanding rather than confrontation. By shifting your perception, you allow yourself to respond with calm and clarity rather than reacting out of fear or defensiveness.

Reframing is a powerful tool because it changes the emotional energy of a situation. Instead of feeling overwhelmed by negativity, you transform the situation into an opportunity for positive action. This shift in mindset is critical for maintaining control in high-stress situations.

3. **Body Regulation**: Our bodies are often the first to react to stress. When we feel anxious, our muscles tense, our heart rate increases, and our posture collapses. Body regulation is about recognizing these physical responses and using techniques to release tension and restore balance.

A powerful body regulation technique is progressive muscle relaxation (PMR). PMR involves tensing and then relaxing different muscle groups in the body to release physical tension. Start by tensing your feet for a few seconds, then releasing them. Move up your body—legs, abdomen, chest, arms, and face—tensing and relaxing each area. This practice helps to reduce physical stress and bring awareness to how the body is responding to emotions.

Additionally, posture plays a key role in how we feel and react. Standing tall with an open chest and shoulders not only makes us appear more confident but also sends signals to our brain that we are in control. Practicing good posture throughout the day helps to keep the body and mind in a state of readiness without the constriction that stress and anxiety can create.

## Conclusion:

Control is a powerful force in our lives, but it's not about dominating the world around us or forcing outcomes. True control lies in mastering ourselves—our reactions, routines, and responses. By reframing our understanding of control and choosing internal power over external force, we can navigate life's challenges with resilience, clarity, and wisdom.

The tactical tools of breathing, reframing, and body regulation give us practical ways to manage high-stress moments and stay in control when emotions run high. These tools help us maintain emotional and mental equilibrium, even when external circumstances are chaotic. When we learn to master ourselves, we become more effective in every area of life—from our relationships to our careers to our health.

The illusion of control can be freeing when we realize that the only thing we truly control is ourselves. By focusing on our own internal mastery, we gain the strength and clarity to navigate life's unpredictable challenges without losing our edge.

# Chapter 5

## The Self-Reliant Toolbox — Building a Mental Fitness Routine

### Introduction:

In this modern world, the concept of mental fitness is becoming increasingly relevant. While physical fitness has long been emphasized as an essential part of a man's well-being, mental fitness is equally crucial for thriving in today's fast-paced, complex environment. However, mental fitness is often seen as a nebulous idea, a concept that is vague and often associated with therapy, journaling, or introspective methods that may not appeal to everyone, particularly those who prefer a more self-reliant, practical approach to personal growth.

This chapter offers a solution to those seeking a more pragmatic way to build and maintain mental resilience—without relying on couches, long therapy sessions, or hours of journaling. The goal is to create a mental fitness routine that can be seamlessly integrated into daily life, one that treats the mind like muscle, builds strength through micro habits, and fosters clarity through intentional reflection. We'll explore how mental conditioning—when done with a systematic approach—can become a transformative and empowering process.

The tools and techniques presented here are simple, straightforward, and highly effective. This isn't about meditative retreats or complex psychological theories. Instead, it's about integrating small, daily practices into your life that promote mental resilience, focus, and self-sufficiency. Think of it as building a "man cave" for your thoughts—a personal space for reflection and growth that doesn't require professional therapy but still offers deep insights and clarity.

By the end of this chapter, you'll have a concrete mental fitness routine that will support your journey toward greater self-reliance, emotional stability, and mental toughness.

## No Couches, No Journals—Just a Plan

While many people turn to therapy or journaling as tools for self-improvement, the reality is that these methods may not work for everyone. Some men might find it difficult to open up to a therapist or sit down with a journal to reflect on their thoughts. The key to mental fitness is not about adopting the methods that others deem effective, but rather creating a plan that aligns with your own style, preferences, and strengths.

Building a mental fitness routine doesn't need to rely on external validation or therapeutic interventions. It's about developing a daily plan that strengthens your mind through intentional practice and consistency. You don't need to "find your inner peace" through long discussions with a therapist, nor do you need to pour your thoughts onto paper to achieve clarity. What you do need is a structure—a plan that is practical, actionable, and works within your busy life.

Think of it like building a fitness regimen for your body. Just as you wouldn't skip leg day or neglect upper body strength, you shouldn't ignore your mental health and clarity. By creating a simple yet effective mental fitness routine, you can build resilience, boost your cognitive abilities, and improve your emotional intelligence—all while focusing on self-reliance and personal growth.

A well-structured plan to develop mental fitness might include daily practices such as maintaining mental clarity, prioritizing sleep, stepping out of your comfort zone, and creating time for solitude. Let's break each of these down to see how they contribute to overall mental strength.

## Mental Conditioning: Treating the Mind Like Muscle

The key to building mental strength is recognizing that, like any other muscle, the mind needs to be conditioned and trained consistently. While physical exercise strengthens the body, mental conditioning strengthens the mind, making it more resilient to stress, adversity, and the challenges life throws at us. The problem is that many people neglect the mental aspects of their well-being, focusing solely on physical health, career success, or material achievement.

Treating the mind like a muscle involves engaging in regular, intentional practices that build cognitive flexibility, emotional resilience, and mental clarity. The more you condition your mind, the stronger it becomes at processing information, making decisions, and managing stress.

- **Cognitive Exercises**: Just as you might lift weights to increase physical strength, there are exercises for the mind that promote mental agility. These can include activities like puzzles, chess, or strategic games that challenge the brain. Reading thought-provoking material and engaging in deep discussions or debates also stimulate mental growth.

- **Mental Toughness Drills**: Mental conditioning also involves strengthening your ability to endure discomfort and persevere in the face of challenges. This could mean pushing through difficult tasks, learning to cope with frustration without losing your composure, or training yourself to stay calm in stressful situations. The more you put yourself in situations that require mental toughness, the more resilient you become.

- **Mindfulness and Focus**: Practicing mindfulness or deep focus on a single task is another form of mental conditioning. Engaging in focused work, whether through meditation or deliberate concentration, trains the mind to resist distractions and improve mental clarity. This is an essential skill in a world filled with constant noise and interruptions.

By treating the mind as a muscle to be trained, you develop the mental stamina necessary to face life's challenges with confidence and resolve. You don't need complex tools or lengthy sessions; what's important is regular, intentional mental conditioning that becomes ingrained in your routine.

## Micro Habits That Create Macro Change (Sleep, Clarity, Challenge, Solitude)

Now that we understand the importance of mental conditioning, the next step is to focus on the micro habits that can lead to macro changes in mental fitness. These habits may seem small, but when practiced consistently, they create significant shifts in your mental and emotional well-being. Let's explore four key micro habits: sleep, clarity, challenge, and solitude.

1. **Sleep**: The foundation of mental clarity and emotional resilience begins with good sleep. Sleep is crucial for memory consolidation, emotional regulation, and cognitive function. Without adequate sleep, our ability to process information, make sound decisions, and manage stress is significantly impaired. Developing a sleep routine is one of the simplest yet most effective micro habits to improve mental fitness.

   o *The Habit*: Set a consistent bedtime and wake-up time, ensuring that you get 7-9 hours of restful sleep each night. Avoid distractions like screens or caffeine before bed, as they can interfere with your ability to fall asleep. Focus on creating an environment that promotes restful sleep—comfortable bedding, a cool room, and limited noise.

   o *Why It Works*: Sleep helps to recharge your brain and body, allowing you to process emotions and stress. Without proper sleep, your mind becomes sluggish, reactive, and less capable of dealing with challenges.

2. **Clarity**: Clarity of thought is essential for making good decisions, staying focused, and effectively managing your emotions. One of the best ways to cultivate mental clarity is by developing the habit of taking moments throughout the day to clear your mind.

   ○ *The Habit*: Set aside time each morning or during the day to engage in a short mental clarity exercise. This could be a few minutes of focused breathing, a quick walk outside, or a short meditation session. The goal is to give your mind a moment to reset, cut through the noise, and bring your focus to the present.

   ○ *Why It Works*: Mental clarity improves cognitive function, decision-making, and emotional regulation. When you take the time to clear your mind, you reduce mental clutter and set yourself up for a more focused, productive day.

3. **Challenge**: Growth happens when we step out of our comfort zone and push ourselves to do things that challenge us. Mental conditioning thrives on tackling new challenges that test our abilities and expand our limits.

   ○ *The Habit*: Identify one area in your life where you can introduce a challenge—whether it's taking on a new project at work, learning a new skill, or pushing yourself physically. This could be as simple as taking a cold shower, running a few extra miles, or learning a new language. The key is to do something that stretches your mental and physical boundaries regularly.

  o  *Why It Works*: Challenges build mental resilience by forcing you to adapt, problem-solve, and overcome obstacles. The more challenges you take on, the stronger your mindset becomes, making you more capable of handling stress, setbacks, and adversity.

4. **Solitude**: Solitude allows for self-reflection, emotional processing, and creative thinking. In a world full of distractions, solitude provides the space for deep thinking and introspection.

  o  *The Habit*: Dedicate time each day or week to being alone with your thoughts. This could mean spending time in nature, taking a solo walk, or engaging in activities that don't require external input, like reading or thinking. The goal is to create space for your mind to roam freely and reflect without distractions.

  o  *Why It Works*: Solitude allows you to connect with yourself and process your emotions, thoughts, and ideas without the influence of others. It promotes self-awareness, creativity, and the ability to think clearly and independently.

By developing these micro habits—prioritizing sleep, cultivating clarity, seeking challenges, and creating time for solitude—you build a foundation for long-term mental fitness. These habits, when practiced consistently, lead to profound changes in how you think, react, and navigate the world.

## Building a "Man Cave" for Thought: A System for Reflection Without Therapy

A "man cave" for thought is a personal, intentional space where you can reflect, recharge, and process your thoughts without the need for therapy or external validation. This space can take many forms, but the idea is simple: create a system for reflection that allows you to gain insights, solve problems, and deepen your self-awareness.

- **The Habit**: Designate a physical or mental space where you can retreat for reflection. This could be a quiet room, a specific chair, or even a daily time slot in your schedule. During this time, allow yourself to think deeply, ask questions, and evaluate your current state. The goal is not to seek answers from others but to engage in self-reflection and mental problem-solving.

- **Why It Works**: Creating a "man cave" for thought allows you to step away from the noise of daily life and engage in deep self-reflection. This space can serve as a personal workshop for your mind, where you can process emotions, clarify your goals, and explore new ideas without distractions.

## Conclusion:

Building mental fitness is a lifelong journey that requires intentionality, consistency, and discipline. By treating the mind like a muscle, developing micro habits that support mental clarity, resilience, and growth, and creating a space for reflection, you can cultivate mental strength and emotional stability. These tools provide a self-reliant path to personal growth, one that doesn't rely on therapy or external support but empowers you to take control of your mental well-being.

The self-reliant toolbox isn't about quick fixes or instant results—it's about laying the groundwork for lasting mental resilience and clarity. By incorporating these practices into your daily life, you'll build a strong, focused mind capable of handling whatever life throws your way. The power to shape your thoughts and your responses is in your hands— master it, and you'll unlock a deeper level of strength, purpose, and self-awareness.

# Chapter 6

## Stoic, Not Stone — Redefining Emotional Resilience

### Introduction:

S ociety often paints a picture of strength as immovable—something that must resist, hold firm, and never bend under pressure. In the modern narrative, emotional resilience is frequently misunderstood as a kind of emotional invulnerability, the ability to endure pain without showing signs of wear. Men are often conditioned to embody this rigid version of strength, where emotions are sidelined, vulnerabilities hidden, and the expectation is to "push through" without revealing any weakness. However, there is a profound wisdom in ancient philosophies, particularly in Stoicism, that suggests the real strength lies not in hardening oneself, but in adapting, bending, and learning from life's challenges.

In this chapter, we will explore the core principles of Stoicism and what it can teach modern men about emotional resilience. Drawing on the wisdom of Marcus Aurelius and other Stoic philosophers, we'll explore how resilience isn't about resistance or being emotionally impervious—it's about adaptability, balance, and developing a mindset that allows us to take hits without hiding or hardening. We'll discuss the idea of emotional "armor that breathes" and how you can develop resilience that doesn't come from stone-like rigidity, but from a flexible, grounded, and reflective approach to life's inevitable challenges.

By the end of this chapter, you will understand how to cultivate emotional resilience in a way that allows you to thrive under pressure, remain calm in adversity, and learn from every experience, no matter how painful.

## What Marcus Aurelius Knew That Modern Men Forgot

Marcus Aurelius, the Roman Emperor and Stoic philosopher, is one of the most enduring figures in the history of philosophy. His *Meditations*—a collection of personal reflections—offer timeless insights into the nature of strength, leadership, and resilience. He wasn't just a powerful ruler; he was a man who wrestled with internal struggles, faced the burdens of leadership, and was deeply committed to self-improvement and emotional balance. Despite the immense power he held, Marcus Aurelius never sought to project an image of invulnerability or to suppress his emotions; instead, he embraced the reality of his humanity, accepting that hardship, loss, and challenges were natural parts of life.

In one of his most famous meditations, Marcus Aurelius writes:

*"The impediment to action advances action. What stands in the way becomes the way."*

This simple yet profound insight holds the key to understanding emotional resilience. Modern men, especially those raised to value toughness above all else, often misunderstand resilience as the ability to avoid pain, discomfort, and vulnerability. We are taught to push forward, no matter the cost. However, Marcus Aurelius recognized that challenges and obstacles are not just things to endure—they are opportunities for growth. The obstacles themselves become the path to greater wisdom, patience, and emotional mastery.

In today's world, we have lost touch with this idea. Many men are taught to reject vulnerability, to resist discomfort, and to "tough it out." But Marcus Aurelius showed us that true resilience isn't about resisting or denying hardship; it's about meeting it with clarity, equanimity, and adaptability.

To modern men, Marcus Aurelius' teachings are a reminder that we don't have to be unfeeling or stoic in the sense of emotional numbness. Rather, we can be resilient by acknowledging our emotions, facing our challenges, and embracing the inevitable hardships of life. The true strength lies not in shutting down our feelings, but in engaging with them intelligently and with purpose.

## Resilience Isn't Resistance—It's Adaptability

One of the greatest misconceptions about resilience is that it requires an unwavering, rigid response to adversity. Society often encourages men to build emotional walls, to bottle up their feelings, and to resist showing any signs of weakness. This form of "resilience" is often framed as the ability to endure without breaking. Yet, what many fail to realize is that true resilience is not about unyielding resistance—it's about adaptability. It's about learning how to bend, adjust, and recalibrate in the face of difficulty, rather than standing firm until the inevitable cracks appear.

Resilience is not about being impervious to life's trials, but about responding to them in ways that promote growth and maintain our mental and emotional equilibrium. This adaptability doesn't mean that we remain unchanged by adversity. On the contrary, it means that we are able to adjust our mindset and approach to life's challenges, learning from them and emerging stronger in the process.

For example, when faced with a difficult situation—whether it's a personal loss, a work setback, or a relationship conflict—resilience might involve acknowledging your pain and then using that emotional experience to reassess your priorities or approach. It could mean reflecting on your response to the situation, adjusting your strategy, or even seeking help from others. Resilience is the ability to stay flexible, not harden yourself against the world.

This adaptability comes from a mindset shift: Instead of viewing challenges as obstacles to be avoided or eliminated, see them as opportunities to grow. It's about learning how to flow with life's changes, finding meaning and purpose in even the most difficult moments. Just as a tree bends in the wind, resilient people bend with the circumstances of their lives, absorbing the impact and emerging stronger rather than breaking under the strain.

## How to Take Hits Without Hiding or Hardening

One of the biggest misconceptions about resilience is that it's synonymous with being unbreakable. The idea of "toughness" often revolves around the notion that you should never show weakness or vulnerability. However, this can lead to emotional suppression, isolation, and an inability to process pain in healthy ways.

The true test of resilience isn't avoiding pain; it's how you respond to it. When you experience emotional blows—whether in the form of failure, loss, criticism, or disappointment—the natural reaction is often to retreat or harden yourself in defense. We may hide our feelings, shut ourselves off from others, or become defensive and aggressive. While these reactions may provide temporary relief, they only prolong suffering and prevent true emotional growth.

To build real emotional resilience, you need to learn how to take hits without retreating into emotional armor or hardening yourself against the world. This requires vulnerability and emotional intelligence—two qualities that are often undervalued in traditional ideas of masculinity. Taking hits without hiding or hardening means allowing yourself to feel the impact of life's challenges, process the emotions that come with them, and then move forward with greater wisdom and purpose.

Here are some ways to take hits without retreating into emotional armor:

1. **Acknowledge Your Emotions**: When faced with adversity, give yourself permission to feel whatever emotions arise. Whether it's anger, sadness, fear, or frustration, these emotions are natural responses to life's challenges. Acknowledging these feelings without judgment allows you to process them in a healthy way.

2. **Reframe the Situation**: As Marcus Aurelius taught, the obstacles in our path can become the way. Reframing a difficult

situation can help you see it as an opportunity for growth, rather than something that's simply blocking your progress. Instead of thinking of failure as something to avoid, see it as an opportunity to learn and improve.

3.  **Seek Support**: Resilience isn't about doing it all alone. It's about knowing when to reach out for support. Whether it's a trusted friend, a mentor, or a support group, having people you can lean on during tough times can help you process your emotions and gain perspective.

4.  **Embrace Self-Compassion**: Instead of criticizing yourself for feeling vulnerable or hurt, practice self-compassion. Understand that it's okay to feel pain, and that these feelings do not define your strength or worth. By treating yourself with kindness during difficult times, you build the emotional capacity to recover and grow.

## The Art of Emotional "Armor that Breathes"

One of the key elements of true emotional resilience is the ability to protect your emotions without shutting them down completely. This concept can be thought of as creating an emotional "armor that breathes"—a defense mechanism that allows you to withstand emotional blows while still remaining connected to your vulnerability and humanity.

Imagine that your emotional armor is not a hard, impenetrable shield but rather a flexible, porous layer that protects you while still allowing air to flow through. This "breathing armor" allows you to absorb the impact of life's challenges without becoming numb or closed off. It gives you the strength to stay engaged with your emotions while also maintaining the resilience to move forward and grow.

The art of emotional armor that breathes involves:

1. **Boundaries**: Healthy emotional boundaries are essential for protecting your emotional well-being without becoming emotionally distant. Boundaries allow you to say no when necessary, protect yourself from toxic influences, and create space for self-care and reflection. Boundaries don't mean shutting yourself off from others; they mean protecting your emotional energy in a way that allows you to engage with the world authentically.

2. **Vulnerability**: Vulnerability is not a weakness; it's a strength. Embracing vulnerability allows you to experience life fully— without the fear of being overwhelmed by emotions. Emotional resilience isn't about suppressing your feelings; it's about learning how to manage them in a way that doesn't consume you. Vulnerability enables connection, empathy, and deeper understanding.

3. **Emotional Regulation**: Building emotional resilience also requires the ability to regulate your emotions in real-time. This doesn't mean suppressing your emotions, but rather understanding and managing them in a way that allows you to stay grounded. Techniques like deep breathing, mindfulness, and

grounding exercises can help you regulate your emotional state in moments of stress or conflict.

4. **Reflection**: Finally, emotional armor that breathes involves regular reflection—taking the time to process your emotions, thoughts, and experiences. This reflection helps you understand what's happening within you, how you're responding to life's challenges, and where you need to adjust. Reflection allows you to heal and grow from your experiences rather than bury them.

## Conclusion:

Emotional resilience is not about building walls to protect yourself from pain—it's about developing the flexibility, strength, and awareness to navigate life's challenges with grace. Stoicism, as exemplified by Marcus Aurelius, teaches us that resilience is not resistance; it's adaptability. By learning how to take hits without hiding or hardening, and by cultivating emotional armor that breathes, we can face adversity with clarity, strength, and purpose.

The journey to emotional resilience is a lifelong process. It requires practice, self-awareness, and the willingness to embrace vulnerability. But when we choose to adapt, learn from hardship, and allow our emotions to be a source of strength rather than weakness, we unlock the true power within ourselves. In the end, emotional resilience is not about avoiding pain—it's about using pain as a catalyst for growth and transformation.

# Chapter 7

# Anger, Burnout, and the Silent Pressure Cooker

## Introduction:

In the world of modern masculinity, emotions like anger are often viewed through a lens of strength, as though they signify a man standing up for himself, asserting dominance, or protecting his territory. However, the truth is more complicated. Anger, for many men, is less about righteous indignation and more about something deeper—an emotional response to pain, frustration, and unprocessed stress. In many cases, what appears as anger is actually a sign of emotional overload, with the root cause often buried under layers of expectations, responsibilities, and unresolved feelings.

On the other hand, burnout is a slow, insidious condition that often affects high-functioning men who are conditioned to keep going no matter the cost. These men don't show the typical signs of burnout—such as neglecting responsibilities or withdrawing from society—but instead push forward, often at the expense of their mental and physical health. This chapter will dive into the connection between anger and burnout, how to recognize the red flags and early warning signs of emotional overload, and how men can find healthy outlets for their emotions before they reach the point of explosive burnout.

By the end of this chapter, you'll understand why anger is often pain in disguise, how burnout can manifest in high-functioning individuals, and how to recognize the signs of emotional overload before it's too late. Most importantly, you'll learn how to turn the pressure valve down and find healthier ways to process and release your emotions.

## Why Anger is Often Pain in Disguise

Anger is often one of the most misunderstood and misdirected emotions. In many cases, anger is not a response to what's happening in the present moment, but rather a reaction to deeper, unaddressed emotional pain. For many men, anger becomes the go-to emotional expression because it is often perceived as stronger or more acceptable than vulnerability, sadness, or fear. It is easier, after all, to be angry than to admit feeling hurt, disappointed, or afraid. Yet, this misplaced expression of emotion can create more harm than good.

Anger often arises when we feel a threat to something we value—whether it's our self-esteem, our ability to succeed, or our sense of control. At its core, anger is a protective emotion that activates when we feel that something is being taken from us, whether it's our dignity, autonomy, or peace of mind. But what many men don't realize is that anger can be a defense mechanism that masks deeper emotions like sadness, shame, fear, or grief.

For example, consider a man who experiences criticism at work. Rather than feeling vulnerable or acknowledging the pain of being judged, he may react with anger, turning the focus away from the discomfort of criticism and toward an outward expression of defiance or frustration. But beneath this reaction, there may be feelings of inadequacy, fear of failure, or shame that have been suppressed and masked by the anger response.

Understanding that anger is often pain in disguise can be transformative. When anger arises, it's important to pause and ask yourself, "What am I truly feeling beneath the surface?" Is there a deeper emotion at play that I'm avoiding? Is this anger a cover-up for feelings of hurt, rejection, or fear?

By acknowledging the root cause of anger—rather than just the surface emotion—you can begin to address the underlying pain, heal the wound, and ultimately express your feelings in healthier, more constructive ways. Instead of letting anger control you, you can learn to understand it, process it, and release it without letting it derail your emotional well-being or relationships.

## What Burnout Looks Like in High-Functioning Men

Burnout is often thought of as something that affects people who are overwhelmed and unable to keep up with their responsibilities. But for high-functioning men, burnout doesn't always look like emotional collapse or withdrawal. In fact, burnout in high-functioning individuals often manifests as overachievement, relentless work, and the appearance of "doing just fine" even as their mental and physical reserves are running dry.

High-functioning burnout is particularly dangerous because it often goes unrecognized until it's too late. These men are typically driven, ambitious, and determined. They may excel in their careers, maintain family obligations, and appear to have it all together. However, beneath the surface, they are struggling to keep up with the constant demands of their lives, leading to a slow erosion of their mental and emotional health.

Here are some key characteristics of burnout in high-functioning men:

- **Chronic Stress**: High-functioning men often experience chronic stress because they are continuously pushing themselves to meet high expectations—whether those expectations come from their jobs, families, or themselves. This constant state of pressure can wear down their mental resources over time, leaving them feeling mentally and emotionally exhausted.

- **Perfectionism**: High-functioning men with burnout often experience perfectionistic tendencies. They feel the need to excel in every aspect of their lives, which leads them to overcommit and overperform. This need for perfection becomes a trap, as it only fuels further stress and emotional exhaustion.

- **Emotional Numbness**: Over time, the constant pressure to perform can lead to emotional detachment. Men experiencing burnout may feel disconnected from their feelings or may suppress their emotions to maintain a façade of control. This emotional numbness often makes it difficult to recognize or address their emotional needs.

- **Physical Symptoms**: Burnout doesn't only affect a person's mental state—it has physical effects as well. High-functioning men may experience frequent headaches, digestive issues, insomnia, or unexplained fatigue. They might ignore these symptoms, dismissing them as normal signs of stress or simply pushing through, but over time, these physical signs of burnout become more pronounced.

- **Impaired Decision Making**: As mental and emotional reserves are depleted, burnout can impair a person's ability to make decisions. What once seemed clear and straightforward becomes muddled by indecision and procrastination. High-functioning individuals may also engage in avoidance behaviors—putting off difficult tasks or failing to prioritize important decisions, leading to further stress.

The key to recognizing burnout in high-functioning men is understanding that it may not look like the conventional image of exhaustion or withdrawal. Instead, it often manifests as a relentless drive to keep going, no matter the cost. If left unchecked, this state can lead to significant emotional and physical damage. Recognizing the signs early is critical to preventing long-term consequences.

## Red Flags and "Early Warnings" of Emotional Overload

There are early warning signs that emotional overload is on the horizon. Just as a pressure cooker builds up steam before it explodes, emotional overload accumulates slowly, often unnoticed, until it becomes too much to handle. Recognizing these red flags early on can help prevent burnout, anger explosions, and other emotional breakdowns.

Some early warning signs include:

1. **Increased Irritability or Short Temper**: When you find yourself getting easily frustrated or snapping at people over minor issues, it may be a sign that you are emotionally overloaded. This irritability is often the result of accumulated stress and frustration that has not been addressed or processed.

2. **Difficulty Sleeping or Restlessness**: Sleep disturbances are one of the most common signs of emotional overload. If you're waking up frequently during the night, struggling to fall asleep, or feeling restless and anxious even when you should be resting, your body is signaling that something is off.

3. **Avoidance or Withdrawal**: If you find yourself withdrawing from social activities, avoiding important conversations, or procrastinating on tasks that you normally would handle, this could be a sign of emotional burnout. Emotional overload often leads to avoidance behaviors, as the mind and body attempt to conserve energy.

4. **Physical Exhaustion Despite Rest**: You may feel tired even after a full night of sleep, or experience ongoing fatigue despite taking breaks. Emotional exhaustion often manifests physically, and when the mind is constantly under stress, it can wear down the body's energy reserves.

5. **Overthinking and Mental Fog**: When you're emotionally overloaded, your brain may become clouded by constant

rumination, worry, and overthinking. This mental fog can make it difficult to focus, make decisions, or complete tasks efficiently.

6. **Frequent Illness or Aches and Pains**: Emotional overload can weaken the immune system, leading to frequent colds, headaches, or digestive issues. Physical symptoms often signal that stress is taking a toll on your body.

7. **Feeling Disconnected or Numb**: As emotional stress builds, you might begin to feel emotionally distant from yourself or others. This emotional numbness is a defense mechanism that the mind uses to protect itself from overwhelming feelings, but it often leads to further disconnection and isolation.

By recognizing these early warning signs, you can take proactive steps to manage emotional overload before it leads to a breakdown. It's important to address these symptoms early on, rather than brushing them aside or pushing through them.

## Healthy Outlets vs. Hidden Explosions

One of the most important aspects of emotional resilience is knowing how to channel your emotions into healthy outlets, rather than allowing them to build up and explode. When men are conditioned to suppress their emotions or bottle up their feelings, they run the risk of reaching a breaking point. This can result in outbursts of anger, emotional breakdowns, or even physical health problems.

Healthy outlets for emotions allow you to process feelings constructively and release emotional pressure before it builds up. Some examples of healthy outlets include:

- **Physical Activity**: Exercise is one of the most effective ways to release built-up emotional tension. Whether through running, weightlifting, yoga, or other forms of movement, physical activity helps reduce stress hormones, improves mood, and provides a healthy release for pent-up emotions.

- **Creative Expression**: Engaging in creative activities such as art, music, writing, or building something tangible provides an emotional release while also fostering a sense of accomplishment and relaxation.

- **Mindfulness and Meditation**: Practicing mindfulness or meditation helps you connect with your emotions in a non-judgmental way, allowing you to process feelings and calm your mind. Even just a few minutes a day can help prevent emotional buildup and promote mental clarity.

- **Talking It Out**: Having honest conversations with trusted friends, family, or mentors can provide emotional relief. Speaking openly about your challenges allows you to gain perspective, feel heard, and receive support.

The key to managing emotions is to establish regular outlets for emotional release, which helps to prevent explosive outbursts. If left unchecked, repressed emotions can cause hidden explosions that damage relationships, health, and personal well-being.

## Conclusion:

Anger, burnout, and emotional overload are real challenges that many men face in today's fast-paced, high-pressure world. By understanding that anger is often pain in disguise, recognizing the early signs of burnout, and learning to find healthy outlets for emotional release, you can take control of your emotional health.

Rather than letting stress, frustration, and unresolved feelings build up like a pressure cooker waiting to explode, you can develop emotional resilience by practicing self-awareness, managing stress proactively, and seeking balance in your life. By confronting your emotions, acknowledging their root causes, and finding ways to release tension before it reaches its breaking point, you can avoid the silent pressure cooker and build a healthier, more sustainable way of coping with life's challenges.

# Chapter 8

# Relationships Without the Drama or Therapy Talk

## Introduction:

Emotions can often feel like a rollercoaster, relationships, especially romantic ones, tend to carry a unique set of challenges. Men are frequently conditioned to believe that in order to connect with others, especially women, they must dive into deep emotional confessions, analyze every feeling, and engage in extensive discussions about vulnerabilities. While emotional openness is undeniably important, the expectation that every relationship must be filled with dramatic conversations or therapy-like exchanges can be exhausting and counterproductive.

This chapter is not about avoiding the depths of emotional connection, but rather about finding a way to connect more authentically and effectively, without being bogged down by drama or over-analyzing every emotion. You'll learn how to communicate with impact, listen like a leader, and navigate relationships with fewer emotional fireworks and more meaningful understanding.

The goal of this chapter is simple: to help you build stronger, healthier relationships by teaching you how to engage with people— especially women—without resorting to therapy talk or overcomplicating things. You'll learn how to speak with clarity, listen effectively, and create emotional space for others without losing yourself in the process.

By the end of this chapter, you'll know how to connect deeply without the drama, understand when to speak, when to fix, and when to simply show up, and most importantly, how to navigate the emotional landscape of relationships without losing your own emotional integrity.

## How to Connect Without Confessing

Many men believe that to form deep, meaningful connections, they must open up about every detail of their emotional world—confessing vulnerabilities, fears, and regrets. While sharing personal experiences can create intimacy, it's important to recognize that genuine connection doesn't always require a deep dive into emotional confession.

In fact, constantly confessing emotions or offering unsolicited vulnerability can sometimes overwhelm others and create unnecessary tension. True emotional connection can be built through simple, honest engagement, shared experiences, and mutual respect, without always needing to spill every emotional detail.

To connect without confessing, consider the following:

1. **Authentic Presence Over Forced Vulnerability**: Emotional intimacy doesn't have to come from over-sharing. Simply being present with someone, showing genuine interest, and engaging in meaningful conversations is often more valuable than confessing every inner feeling. When you're truly present—listening intently,

observing body language, and being mindful of the moment— you build rapport and understanding without needing to confess.

2. **Shared Activities Over Verbal Confessions**: Engaging in activities together is often more powerful than sitting down for a "confession session." Whether it's cooking a meal, going for a hike, or working on a shared project, these activities allow you to connect without necessarily delving into your deepest emotions. Shared experiences provide a natural space for emotional connection to develop, without the need for constant emotional disclosures.

3. **Let Actions Speak Louder Than Words**: Sometimes, emotional connection is best communicated through action rather than conversation. When you offer support, express care, and provide comfort in the small, everyday ways, it creates a foundation of trust and intimacy. You don't need to constantly confess or verbalize your emotions to show that you care—your actions will do the talking.

Connecting without confessing doesn't mean you avoid being emotionally open. Instead, it means recognizing that relationships are built on mutual understanding and respect, which can grow through shared moments and genuine interaction, rather than through forced emotional disclosures.

# Listening Like a Leader: High-Impact Communication Without Fluff

Listening is one of the most underrated, yet most powerful, tools in building strong relationships. Unfortunately, many men are taught to listen with the intention of fixing, offering solutions, or "getting to the point" as quickly as possible. This style of communication often misses the nuance and depth of the other person's experience.

To truly connect, especially in intimate relationships, listening must go beyond just hearing words; it requires emotional engagement, focus, and leadership. "Listening like a leader" is about being present in the conversation, paying attention to the emotional landscape of the speaker, and providing a safe space for them to express themselves without judgment or interruption.

Here's how to practice high-impact listening without fluff:

1. **Listen with Intention**: Instead of passively hearing what the other person is saying, actively listen with the intent to understand. Avoid the urge to interrupt or immediately offer advice. Instead, focus on what they're feeling, what they might not be saying, and the underlying emotions behind their words. High-impact listening allows you to grasp the full context, which helps you respond thoughtfully.

2. **Empathy Over Problem-Solving**: One of the most common mistakes in relationships, especially for men, is the impulse to fix problems rather than just listen. While offering solutions is sometimes necessary, it's not always the right response. Often,

people—particularly women—just want to be heard and understood. Instead of jumping in with your solutions, try offering empathy first. Validate their feelings by saying things like, "I can understand why you feel that way," or "That sounds really challenging." This shows emotional maturity and leadership in communication.

3. **Ask Clarifying Questions**: Great leaders ask insightful questions that deepen the conversation and encourage the other person to explore their feelings. Rather than offering opinions, ask questions that encourage deeper reflection and open up the dialogue. Questions like "How did that make you feel?" or "What was going through your mind when that happened?" give the speaker the space to explore their emotions further and foster a stronger connection.

4. **Non-Verbal Communication**: Listening isn't just about what you say—it's also about how you physically engage with the conversation. Use body language that shows you're fully present: maintain eye contact, nod occasionally to show understanding, and avoid distractions like checking your phone. Your physical presence conveys interest, care, and respect.

By listening with this leadership mindset, you can foster more meaningful communication that strengthens relationships and deepens emotional intimacy.

# When to Speak, When to Fix, and When to Just Show Up

One of the most challenging aspects of relationships, especially romantic ones, is knowing when to speak, when to offer solutions, and when to simply show up and be present. Many men, conditioned by society's emphasis on problem-solving, tend to lean toward fixing issues as soon as they arise. However, not every situation requires a solution, and sometimes the best thing you can do is just be there, listening and offering your presence.

Here's a simple breakdown of when to speak, when to fix, and when to just show up:

1.  **When to Speak**: Speak when your words can provide clarity, support, or encouragement. Sometimes, verbal communication is needed to address misunderstandings or provide reassurance. Offering a gentle, thoughtful comment when necessary can show that you're engaged and invested in the relationship. However, always ensure that your words are rooted in empathy and respect. Avoid speaking just to fill silence or because you feel obligated to say something.

2.  **When to Fix**: Offer solutions only when the other person explicitly asks for them or when you can see that your input will genuinely help resolve the issue. Offering unsolicited advice can often come across as dismissive, as though the other person's emotions or perspective don't matter. Focus on asking questions

to help the person arrive at their own conclusions, which will often be more empowering than simply giving them the answer.

3. **When to Just Show Up**: The most profound moments in relationships often don't require speaking or fixing at all. Sometimes, the most meaningful thing you can do is just show up—physically and emotionally—without any agenda. Whether it's offering a comforting touch, sitting in silence together, or just being there while the other person processes their emotions, your presence can be the most valuable gift. It shows that you are reliable and supportive, even when there's nothing to "fix."

Understanding the balance between speaking, fixing, and simply showing up is a powerful tool in maintaining healthy, drama-free relationships. It allows you to engage in a way that honors the needs of both you and your partner, creating an atmosphere of trust and understanding.

## Navigating Women's Emotional World Without Losing Your Own

One of the most complex aspects of relationships, particularly for men, is understanding how to navigate the emotional world of women without losing your own emotional stability. Women often experience emotions more intensely, and societal expectations encourage them to express and communicate these feelings openly. As a result, men can sometimes feel overwhelmed or unsure of how to engage with their partner's emotional world without getting caught up in it or losing themselves.

Here are some key strategies for navigating women's emotional world while maintaining your own balance:

1. **Understand Emotional Expression vs. Emotional Reaction**: Women may express their emotions differently from men, and this can sometimes create misunderstandings. While men might be more solution-oriented, women might express their emotions as a form of communication or connection, not necessarily seeking a fix. Recognize that when a woman shares her emotions, she is often seeking validation and understanding, not necessarily a solution. Responding with empathy—acknowledging her feelings without feeling the need to immediately fix the situation—can help you navigate her emotional world without getting lost in it.

2. **Stay Grounded in Your Own Emotions**: While it's important to engage with and understand your partner's feelings, don't lose sight of your own emotional landscape. Keep yourself grounded and maintain your emotional boundaries. If you feel overwhelmed by her emotions, take a moment to recalibrate. Practice self-regulation techniques like deep breathing or stepping back for a brief moment to maintain clarity.

3. **Communicate Your Boundaries**: It's essential to communicate your own emotional boundaries respectfully and clearly. If you feel like a conversation is becoming too emotionally charged or draining, it's okay to set limits. You can say something like, "I understand that this is important, but I need a few minutes to

process before we continue." Setting boundaries isn't about shutting her down, but rather about protecting your emotional well-being while still being supportive.

4. **Be an Active Supporter, Not a Fixer**: When women express intense emotions, your role isn't to solve the problem immediately or try to make everything better. Instead, focus on being an active listener and a supportive partner. Ask her how you can best support her in that moment, whether it's through a hug, a reassuring word, or just your undivided attention.

By understanding how to navigate a woman's emotional world while maintaining your own emotional integrity, you can foster a deeper, more connected relationship. You don't have to sacrifice your own emotional health to be a good partner; instead, find ways to honor both your feelings and hers in a balanced, respectful manner.

## Conclusion:

Building relationships without the drama or therapy talk requires understanding, self-awareness, and effective communication. Connecting without confessing, listening like a leader, knowing when to speak, fix, or simply show up, and navigating the emotional world of others without losing your own integrity are all key components of healthy, drama-free relationships.

By focusing on meaningful, authentic communication and emotional balance, you can cultivate deeper connections that are rooted in mutual respect, trust, and understanding—without the need for constant emotional analysis or dramatic exchanges. Relationships are meant to enhance our lives, not drain them. By applying these principles, you can create relationships that are not only fulfilling but also free of unnecessary conflict and emotional turbulence.

# Chapter 9

# Brotherhood and Real Bonds (Beyond Beer and Ballgames)

## Introduction:

Men are often encouraged to focus on career success, personal achievements, and family responsibilities; friendships—particularly male friendships—can sometimes take a back seat. While many men may have experienced a sense of camaraderie and connection during their younger years—through sports, shared interests, or social activities—these relationships can often fade as adulthood sets in. The demands of work, family, and personal growth can lead to a gradual distancing from friends, leaving men feeling isolated or disconnected, even as they continue to succeed in other areas of their lives.

But male friendships are not only about shared experiences like beer, ballgames, or mutual hobbies. True brotherhood—the kind that sustains men through life's challenges and triumphs—is based on trust, emotional support, and an understanding that transcends superficial connections. The problem, however, is that many men don't know how to nurture and sustain deep friendships as they grow older. Emotional vulnerability, which is often undervalued in traditional masculine norms, can be seen as a weakness rather than a strength.

This chapter aims to explore the complex dynamics of male friendships and provide strategies for building and maintaining genuine bonds. We'll look at why adult male friendships often fade, the untapped value of emotional alliances, how to build trust without oversharing, and how strong men support each other in ways that are often silent but profoundly powerful.

By the end of this chapter, you will understand how to reconnect with the deep value of brotherhood, rebuild meaningful friendships, and create a network of strong emotional alliances that support your personal growth and well-being.

## Why Adult Male Friendships Fade—and How to Get Them Back

As men transition from adolescence to adulthood, life often becomes more complicated. Careers, relationships, and family obligations take priority, leaving little time or energy for maintaining the friendships that were once a core part of life. Adult male friendships often fade for several reasons, and understanding these dynamics is key to rebuilding and strengthening these bonds.

1. **Time and Priorities**: In early adulthood, socializing with friends often comes naturally. But as life becomes busier with career advancement, family responsibilities, and personal commitments, time spent with friends becomes scarce. The pressures of adult life can leave little room for the unstructured hangouts or spontaneous outings that once defined friendships. Men, often

focusing on their roles as providers and achievers, may neglect the emotional nourishment that friendships offer.

2. **Shifting Interests**: Over time, people's interests and priorities evolve. The sports bar gatherings and casual hangouts of youth may no longer hold the same appeal once men enter new stages of their lives. Different lifestyles, hobbies, or values can create unspoken gaps between friends, making it harder to maintain common ground.

3. **Emotional Distance**: Unlike women, who are often socialized to maintain close-knit, emotionally expressive relationships, men may find it difficult to share their deeper feelings or vulnerabilities. As a result, friendships may become surface-level or transactional—based on mutual hobbies, work, or casual encounters rather than emotional connection. The inability to communicate emotionally or to offer support during difficult times can gradually erode the strength of these friendships.

4. **Fear of Vulnerability**: In many cultures, men are conditioned to be self-reliant and strong, which can make it difficult to admit emotional needs or struggles. This cultural script leads many men to shut down emotionally, even with close friends. Without the willingness to be vulnerable, friendships become shallow, and emotional distance begins to grow.

So, how can men revive these faded friendships? The answer lies in prioritizing connection and shifting the focus away from superficial bonding toward more meaningful, emotionally supportive interactions. Here's how:

1. **Reach Out**: The first step in rebuilding a friendship is simply reaching out. In today's world, it's easy for life to get in the way of making the effort, but reconnecting with old friends requires taking initiative. A simple message or invitation to meet up can be the catalyst to rekindle a meaningful bond.

2. **Make Time for Friendship**: Even amidst busy schedules, make a conscious effort to schedule regular time with your friends. Whether it's a weekly phone call, a monthly dinner, or a spontaneous weekend trip, setting aside time for your friends ensures that your bond remains strong.

3. **Prioritize Emotional Connection**: Rather than only engaging in activities like watching sports or grabbing a drink, make an effort to talk about more meaningful topics—career challenges, personal goals, or life struggles. Sharing these moments of vulnerability helps deepen your connection and builds a foundation of trust.

4. **Be Consistent**: Friendships require consistent effort to grow and evolve. Small gestures of care—checking in with a friend during tough times, offering support, or celebrating achievements—go a long way in maintaining long-lasting bonds.

## The Underestimated Value of Male Emotional Alliances

Men are often taught to keep their emotions in check and avoid expressing vulnerability, which can create a significant emotional void in their lives. As a result, many men miss out on the invaluable support that comes from strong emotional alliances. Emotional support is often relegated to intimate partners or family, while friendships are viewed through the lens of shared activities and interests. This underestimates the power of having close male friendships where emotions can be freely shared and understood.

The truth is, men who have close emotional alliances with other men experience numerous benefits:

1. **Increased Emotional Resilience**: Having a trusted male friend to confide in during difficult times provides a sense of emotional security. This helps men navigate personal challenges, including stress, relationship issues, and career setbacks. Emotional support from a friend can reduce feelings of isolation and increase resilience, making it easier to cope with adversity.

2. **Better Mental Health**: Emotional alliances have been shown to improve mental health by providing a sense of belonging and reducing feelings of loneliness. Men who have close friendships are less likely to suffer from depression and anxiety because they have people with whom they can share their struggles and triumphs.

3. **Social Bonding and Strengthened Identity**: Strong male friendships provide an opportunity for social bonding that fosters

a sense of shared identity and purpose. These alliances allow men to explore different aspects of themselves, challenge each other, and grow in a way that strengthens their social bonds and personal growth.

4. **A Safe Space for Vulnerability**: When men build emotional alliances, they create safe spaces where vulnerability is welcomed, not judged. Being able to express fear, frustration, or sadness in a non-judgmental environment fosters deeper connections and helps men develop emotional intelligence.

5. **Role Models for Healthy Relationships**: Emotional alliances between men set an example for how to build healthy relationships based on mutual respect, trust, and understanding. These friendships can also serve as models for men on how to navigate romantic or familial relationships with empathy and emotional depth.

Building these emotional alliances requires that men actively choose to show up for each other—not just in good times, but especially when things get tough. It's about offering support when needed and allowing oneself to be vulnerable enough to receive support in return.

## How to Build Trust Without Oversharing

Trust is the foundation of any strong friendship, but many men struggle with the idea of building trust without oversharing personal details or emotional burdens. Oversharing can often feel like a shortcut to creating intimacy, but it can also overwhelm the other person and may create unnecessary pressure. Building trust in a friendship doesn't require oversharing; it requires consistency, reliability, and understanding.

Here's how to build trust without oversharing:

1. **Be Reliable and Consistent**: Trust is built over time through consistent actions. Showing up for your friend, being there during difficult times, and following through on commitments creates a strong foundation of trust. Being consistent in your words and actions ensures that your friend knows they can count on you.

2. **Respect Boundaries**: Trust isn't just about sharing secrets or personal experiences. It's also about respecting each other's boundaries. Knowing when to listen, when to speak, and when to give your friend space is key to maintaining trust in the relationship.

3. **Demonstrate Emotional Support**: Trust is also built by showing empathy and understanding. You don't need to overshare to show your friend that you care. Sometimes, simply listening without judgment, offering a kind word, or being there during tough moments can create a deeper sense of trust than any amount of confessional dialogue.

4. **Be Authentic, Not Perfect**: Trust grows from authenticity. You don't need to share every part of your emotional world to be real with your friends. Simply being honest and showing up as your true self—without pretending to be perfect or constantly seeking approval—creates an environment where trust can flourish.

5. **Create Emotional Safety**: Trust thrives when men feel emotionally safe with each other. This means creating an environment where both of you can express vulnerability, admit weaknesses, and share personal struggles without fear of judgment or rejection. When men create emotionally safe spaces for each other, trust deepens naturally.

## The Silent Support System: How Strong Men Back Each Other

One of the most powerful aspects of male friendship is the silent support system that exists between close friends. This system doesn't rely on constant words of affirmation or overt displays of emotion, but rather on a deep, unspoken understanding that you've got each other's backs—no matter what.

Strong men often back each other in subtle, silent ways. This might include:

1. **Checking In Without Saying Anything**: Sometimes, the most powerful support comes in the form of a simple text or phone call saying, "Hey, I'm thinking of you," without needing to go into great detail. The unspoken message is clear: "I'm here for you, and I care."

2. **Providing Space When Needed**: Silent support often involves understanding when your friend needs space and allowing them to take the time they need. There's no pressure to talk or explain

anything—just knowing that you're there if and when they need you can be incredibly supportive.

3. **Being There in Times of Crisis**: During moments of personal crisis or stress, a strong male friendship shows itself through action. Offering help without expectation, such as showing up when your friend needs assistance, lending a hand when life becomes overwhelming, or providing financial or emotional support in times of need, demonstrates silent strength.

4. **Celebrating Each Other's Successes**: Men often show support by acknowledging and celebrating each other's achievements, both big and small. A simple word of recognition or encouragement can strengthen the bond between friends and reinforce the feeling that success is meant to be shared.

5. **Offering Unspoken Reassurance**: Often, the best way to back your friend is simply through unspoken reassurance. A gesture like a knowing look, a gentle nod, or standing side by side without saying a word can communicate that your friendship remains solid, no matter what challenges arise.

These forms of silent support create a foundation of strength, trust, and mutual respect. They allow men to support each other without overburdening each other with words or constant emotional labor.

## Conclusion:

Brotherhood and genuine emotional bonds between men are often undervalued and underexplored in society. Yet, these relationships—

when built on trust, emotional support, and mutual respect—are a vital source of strength, resilience, and personal growth. By understanding why adult male friendships fade, appreciating the value of emotional alliances, learning to build trust without oversharing, and recognizing the silent support system that exists between strong men, you can foster deeper, more meaningful connections that enhance your emotional well-being.

Building and maintaining brotherhood is not about constant confessions, but about showing up for each other in authentic, reliable ways. True connection is forged in the quiet moments of support, the shared experiences, and the commitment to being present for one another. By prioritizing these elements, men can reclaim the power of true brotherhood and create lasting, emotionally rich relationships that stand the test of time.

# Chapter 10

# Focus, Purpose, and the War Against Distraction

## Introduction:

We are constantly surrounded by distractions. From the endless streams of notifications pinging on our phones to the 24/7 demands of work, social media, and the general noise of modern life, staying focused and maintaining a clear sense of purpose has never been harder. The culture of "always on" has become an inescapable reality for many men, leading to mental fatigue, decreased productivity, and a sense of being overwhelmed by the sheer volume of external stimuli.

Men, in particular, are increasingly struggling with how to manage these distractions effectively while still maintaining their focus on what matters most. The rise of digital devices, the obsession with instant gratification, and the constant barrage of information have created a mental load that can be difficult to manage. Yet, amidst this chaos, the ability to cultivate focus, develop discipline, and maintain a strong sense of purpose is more important than ever before.

This chapter will explore the mental load caused by the "always on" culture, the dopamine traps that keep us hooked on distractions, and how men often numb themselves instead of processing emotions and challenges. We will also delve into the discipline of focus—discussing how routines, rituals, and reason can help men reclaim control over their attention and energy. Lastly, we'll look at how purpose serves as the anchor for a stormy life, providing the clarity and drive necessary to cut through the noise and focus on what truly matters.

By the end of this chapter, you will have a clearer understanding of how to navigate the distractions of modern life, enhance your ability to focus, and use purpose as a guiding principle to lead a more intentional, fulfilling life.

## The Mental Load of "Always On" Culture

The rise of technology, combined with the ever-expanding demands of work, has given birth to a culture that's always on. We're constantly expected to be available, to respond quickly, and to engage with the endless flow of information that surrounds us. This relentless connectivity has created a mental load that is unprecedented—our minds are now tasked with managing multiple streams of communication, decision-making, and emotional responses all at once.

This "always on" culture can be incredibly draining, especially for men who are trying to balance career, family, and personal growth. While technology offers immense convenience, it also creates an environment where the boundaries between work and personal life become increasingly blurred. Emails, messages, social media updates, and other digital noise constantly demand our attention, leaving little space for deep focus or relaxation.

The effects of this mental load are profound. Research has shown that constantly switching between tasks or attempting to multitask can reduce productivity, increase stress levels, and lead to burnout. Our brains are not wired to handle continuous input from external sources without adequate breaks. Over time, this constant bombardment of information can cause cognitive fatigue, reduce our ability to think clearly, and lead to a general feeling of being overwhelmed.

For many men, the inability to escape the "always on" culture leads to mental exhaustion. The need to be constantly available can make it difficult to disconnect, relax, or focus on the tasks that matter most. The mental load, when left unchecked, results in burnout, emotional depletion, and an inability to concentrate on the things that truly bring fulfillment.

## Dopamine Traps, Digital Noise, and How Men Numb Instead of Process

In addition to the constant mental load, modern technology and digital culture create dopamine traps that keep us hooked on distractions. Dopamine, the neurotransmitter associated with pleasure and reward, is triggered every time we check our phones, refresh social media, or respond to a text message. These small, quick rewards provide instant gratification, but at a cost. The more we engage with these distractions, the more we train our brains to crave them. This leads to a cycle of addictive behavior, where we constantly seek out new sources of stimulation, without ever allowing ourselves the space to pause and reflect.

For men, this addiction to instant gratification can lead to emotional numbing. Rather than processing emotions, challenges, or frustrations, many men turn to digital distractions—social media, video games, streaming platforms, and other forms of digital entertainment—as a way to avoid confronting their feelings. This numbing behavior can temporarily alleviate emotional pain or discomfort, but it ultimately prevents men from engaging with their emotions in a meaningful way.

Numbing emotions through digital distractions creates a barrier to emotional growth and self-awareness. Instead of addressing the underlying issues that lead to stress or anxiety, men may choose to escape into the immediate pleasure of their devices. Over time, this avoidance leads to a deeper sense of dissatisfaction and disconnection from one's own feelings. It also makes it more difficult to develop emotional resilience and work through life's challenges with clarity and purpose.

Breaking free from this cycle requires conscious effort and self-awareness. It means learning to resist the pull of dopamine traps and finding healthier outlets for emotional processing. Rather than numbing oneself with distractions, men need to learn how to sit with their feelings, confront their challenges, and develop emotional intelligence. Only then can they reclaim their focus and sense of control.

## The Discipline of Focus: Routine, Ritual, and Reason

In a world full of distractions, the ability to focus is a rare and valuable skill. But focus is not something that comes naturally—it must be cultivated through discipline, routine, and intentional practice. Just as physical fitness requires consistent effort to build strength, mental fitness requires the development of habits that support focus and clarity.

1. **Routine**: Establishing a daily routine is one of the most effective ways to improve focus. When you create a predictable structure for your day, you eliminate decision fatigue and free up mental energy for more important tasks. A well-structured routine sets the tone for the day, providing a sense of purpose and direction. It also helps to build momentum, as completing small tasks early in the day creates a sense of accomplishment that fuels motivation for larger challenges.

   o *How to Build a Routine*: Start by identifying the most important tasks you need to accomplish each day. Block out time in your schedule for these tasks and make them a non-negotiable part of your routine. Incorporate activities that support mental clarity and well-being— such as exercise, meditation, or reading—into your daily practice. Consistency is key. The more you stick to your routine, the more natural focus will become.

2. **Ritual**: Rituals are a powerful way to anchor focus and create a sense of purpose in your life. A ritual is an intentional, meaningful activity that you do regularly, and it can serve as a mental cue to transition into a state of deep focus. Rituals can be simple—like a morning coffee, a walk, or a few minutes of mindfulness—but they provide a structured way to signal your brain that it's time to shift into productive mode.

○ *How to Create Rituals*: Think about the activities that help you feel centered, calm, and focused. This might include a brief stretching routine, a meditation practice, or journaling. You can also create rituals around work, such as dedicating the first 30 minutes of your day to deep work, free from distractions. Rituals create a sense of intention and purpose that enhances your ability to stay focused.

3. **Reason**: Focus requires clarity of purpose. Without a clear reason for why you're doing something, it's easy to get distracted or lose motivation. Having a strong sense of reason provides a guiding principle that anchors your actions. Whether it's a long-term career goal, a personal development objective, or a relationship you're working to improve, knowing why you're dedicating time and energy to a task helps maintain focus and drive.

○ *How to Cultivate Reason*: Take time to reflect on your values and long-term goals. What do you want to achieve in life, and why is it important to you? Write down your core objectives and keep them visible, so they serve as a reminder of your purpose. When distractions arise, revisit your reason for pursuing your goals, and use it to fuel your determination.

Developing the discipline of focus is about creating the right environment for mental clarity and staying intentional with your time and energy. By establishing a routine, incorporating rituals that signal focus, and grounding your actions in a strong sense of reason, you can reclaim your attention and improve your ability to focus on what matters most.

## Purpose as the Anchor for a Stormy Life

In the midst of a world that's constantly pulling for our attention, it's easy to get lost in the noise and lose sight of what really matters. Without a clear sense of purpose, life can feel directionless, and distractions can easily derail us. Purpose is the anchor that keeps us grounded, providing the clarity and motivation needed to navigate the stormy waters of life.

1. **Purpose as a Guiding Light**: Having a strong sense of purpose gives you a reason to keep going, even when the going gets tough. It helps you prioritize your time, energy, and efforts toward something meaningful. When you have a clear purpose, you're more likely to make decisions that align with your values and goals, rather than being swayed by external pressures or distractions.

2. **Purpose Provides Emotional Resilience**: Life is filled with challenges, setbacks, and unexpected changes. Purpose acts as an emotional anchor during these times, reminding you of your long-term goals and helping you stay focused on what matters most. When you face adversity, your purpose gives you the strength to push through difficulties and stay aligned with your vision.

3. **Purpose Drives Motivation**: Without purpose, it's easy to become complacent, lose momentum, or get sidetracked by

distractions. Purpose fuels motivation by providing a reason to keep moving forward. Whether it's a personal achievement, a career milestone, or a desire to help others, your purpose serves as the driving force behind your actions and decisions.

4. **Aligning with Your Purpose**: To harness the power of purpose, take time to identify what truly matters to you. What do you want to contribute to the world? What legacy do you want to leave? Clarifying your purpose allows you to create a roadmap for your life and make decisions that align with your values. When you have a clear sense of purpose, you can navigate life's distractions with greater ease, maintaining focus on the things that truly bring fulfillment.

Purpose is the bedrock of focus. It provides direction, motivation, and emotional resilience in the face of life's inevitable storms. By connecting with your deeper sense of purpose, you can cut through the noise and stay anchored in what truly matters.

## Conclusion:

The battle against distraction in the "always on" culture is one that many men are fighting daily. But through the discipline of focus, the creation of meaningful routines, rituals, and reason, and the anchoring power of purpose, men can reclaim their attention, energy, and emotional resilience. By learning to manage the mental load of modern life, resist dopamine traps, and stay connected to what truly matters, men can create a life of intentionality and fulfillment, regardless of the distractions that surround them.

Focus, purpose, and discipline are the antidotes to the chaos of modern life. By cultivating these qualities, you can build a life that is grounded, purposeful, and immune to the noise and distractions that threaten to derail your journey. The battle for focus is not just a battle for productivity—it's a battle for clarity, meaning, and the ability to live life on your own terms.

# Chapter 11

# Stress Without the Spiral — Handling Pressure Like a Pro

## Introduction:

Stress is a natural part of life. Whether you're facing a looming deadline, managing a high-stakes project, or navigating personal challenges, pressure is something we all experience. However, how we respond to that stress can make the difference between thriving and spiraling into overwhelm. For many men, especially those in high-pressure environments—be it the military, athletics, or the corporate world—the ability to manage stress effectively is not only a necessity but a critical skill that separates high performers from those who falter under pressure.

The ability to handle stress without falling into a mental spiral is one of the most valuable skills you can develop. It's not about eliminating stress, but about managing it in a way that enhances your performance rather than hindering it. This chapter will explore strategies from high-performing men—military personnel, athletes, executives—and provide practical tools to help you handle stress like a pro. We'll dive into crisis management tactics, techniques like tactical breathing and box thinking, and how to stay rational under fire using the logic-emotion handshake.

You'll learn when to push through, when to pivot, and when to pause to ensure that you are making the best possible decisions under pressure.

By the end of this chapter, you'll have a set of actionable tools and insights to turn stress from a source of anxiety into a driving force for success.

## Crisis Management Tactics from High-Performing Men (Military, Athletes, Executives)

When we think of high-performing individuals, we often think of those who excel under pressure: soldiers in the military, top athletes, and high-level executives. All of these individuals operate in environments where stress is a constant companion, yet they seem to navigate it with a level of poise and composure that most people can only dream of. How do they do it?

1. **Military Tactics**: In the military, stress management is not just a skill—it's a matter of life and death. Soldiers are trained to perform under extreme pressure, where the consequences of failure can be catastrophic. One key element of military training is teaching individuals to break down complex problems into smaller, more manageable tasks. Soldiers use crisis management techniques like "combat breathing," focusing on the task at hand, and maintaining mental clarity by sticking to predefined protocols.

   o **Principle of "Mindfulness under Pressure"**: In a combat situation, the military teaches soldiers to remain present and focused, blocking out distractions that can cause panic or confusion. This is achieved through a combination of training, physical conditioning, and mental rehearsals, so soldiers can act decisively when under pressure, without letting fear or anxiety cloud their judgment.

○ **The Importance of Teamwork**: In high-stress military situations, the focus is not just on individual performance but also on teamwork. Soldiers rely on each other, knowing that the support of their peers can make the difference between success and failure. This sense of camaraderie and shared responsibility enables military personnel to face stress with a sense of solidarity and shared purpose.

2. **Athletes' Approach to Stress**: Professional athletes are no strangers to high-pressure situations. Whether it's making a game-winning shot or competing for a gold medal, athletes are often under immense pressure to perform. The key to handling stress in these situations lies in mental conditioning, preparation, and emotional control.

○ **Visualization and Mental Rehearsal**: Many athletes use visualization techniques to prepare for high-pressure situations. By mentally rehearsing the scenario before it happens, athletes create a sense of familiarity and control, which reduces anxiety. This technique allows athletes to feel more confident when the moment arrives because they've already "seen" themselves succeed under pressure.

- ○ **Focused Attention**: Athletes also train their minds to stay focused on the present moment. Instead of letting the pressure of the situation cloud their judgment, they focus on the next step, the next play, or the next move. This approach keeps them grounded and ensures that they are taking one step at a time, rather than getting overwhelmed by the bigger picture.

3. **Executive Crisis Management**: Executives often face pressure in the form of tight deadlines, high stakes decisions, and complex problems that impact entire organizations. The ability to remain calm and make rational decisions in such situations is crucial. High-performing executives manage stress by relying on structured decision-making processes, risk assessments, and clear communication.

- ○ **Decision Frameworks**: Successful executives often use decision-making frameworks to cut through the noise and make informed choices quickly. By breaking down complex problems into smaller components and evaluating options based on data and logic, they can stay calm and make sound decisions, even when under pressure.

○ **Delegation and Trust**: A key strategy for executives is delegating tasks and trusting their team to handle certain responsibilities. This reduces the mental load on the executive and allows them to focus on the bigger picture. High-performing leaders understand that they cannot do everything themselves and rely on their teams to carry out tasks efficiently and effectively.

## Tools: Tactical Breathing, Box Thinking, Decision Anchors

Handling stress like a pro requires more than just a mindset shift—it requires practical tools that can help you stay grounded, focused, and in control. Here are some of the most effective tools used by high performers to manage stress and pressure:

1. **Tactical Breathing**: One of the most powerful techniques for managing stress in high-pressure situations is tactical breathing. Used by military personnel, first responders, and athletes alike, this technique involves slowing down the breath to activate the parasympathetic nervous system, which helps to calm the body and mind.

   ○ **4-4-8 Breathing Technique**: This technique involves inhaling for a count of 4, holding your breath for 4, and then exhaling slowly for a count of 8. By focusing on your breath and regulating the rhythm, you can lower your heart rate, reduce anxiety, and improve mental clarity.

This simple practice can be done in moments of stress to quickly regain focus and control.

2. **Box Thinking**: Box thinking is a mental model that helps you break down complex problems into smaller, more manageable tasks. It involves creating a "box" in your mind that represents the current issue or challenge, and then isolating specific aspects of the problem within that box. This helps you to focus on what can be controlled, while reducing the overwhelming nature of the situation.

   o **How to Apply Box Thinking**: When facing a challenging situation, take a few moments to mentally "box" the problem. Identify key components of the issue and prioritize them. Tackle one problem at a time, instead of allowing yourself to be overwhelmed by the larger situation. This process helps you stay focused on immediate, actionable steps, rather than getting lost in the complexity of the entire scenario.

3. **Decision Anchors**: Decision anchors are mental guides that help you make decisions more quickly and confidently, even in high-pressure situations. They are based on your core values, long-term goals, and predefined rules for decision-making. When faced with a difficult choice, decision anchors help you stay grounded in your principles, reducing the mental strain of indecision and uncertainty.

○ **Creating Decision Anchors**: To create your own decision anchors, reflect on your values and long-term objectives. What is most important to you? What principles guide your decisions? When faced with a high-pressure situation, refer back to these anchors to make decisions that align with your core values, rather than being swayed by external pressures or emotional reactions.

## Staying Rational Under Fire: The Logic-Emotion Handshake

One of the greatest challenges in high-pressure situations is managing the balance between logic and emotion. Emotions are natural responses to stress, but they can cloud judgment and lead to impulsive decisions. On the other hand, pure logic without emotional consideration can make you seem cold, detached, or disconnected from the reality of the situation.

The "logic-emotion handshake" is the ability to balance both of these forces. It involves acknowledging your emotions—whether it's fear, anxiety, or frustration—without allowing them to dictate your actions. At the same time, it's about using logical thinking and analysis to guide your decision-making, ensuring that your emotions don't lead you to act rashly or impulsively.

▪ **How to Achieve the Logic-Emotion Handshake**: Start by acknowledging your emotional response to a situation. It's important to recognize what you're feeling and why, without judgment. Then, take a step back and evaluate the situation using logic and reason. Ask yourself: What is the best course of action based on the facts at hand? What outcome am I aiming for? By balancing both emotion and logic, you can make decisions that are grounded in reality, while also respecting your emotional needs.

## When to Push, When to Pivot, When to Pause

Knowing when to push forward, when to pivot, and when to pause is critical for managing stress effectively. These decisions are often not easy, but understanding when to take action and when to step back can determine the outcome of a high-pressure situation.

1. **When to Push**: Push forward when you have a clear direction, your objectives are aligned with your goals, and you have the mental and physical resources to continue. Pushing forward is appropriate when you are in a position to act decisively and confidently, and when the situation demands swift action.

   o **Indicators to Push**: Clear priorities, a sense of urgency, and confidence in your ability to execute. If there's an opportunity for momentum and the potential for success is high, pushing forward can build momentum and keep things moving.

2. **When to Pivot**: Pivot when you realize that the current approach isn't working, or when new information arises that changes the course of action. Pivoting is necessary when staying the course

would lead to inefficiency, failure, or unnecessary stress. It's about being adaptable and open to adjusting your strategy when the situation calls for it.

- ○ **Indicators to Pivot**: New data or insights, failure to achieve progress, changing circumstances, or an emotional signal that the current path is no longer sustainable. A pivot is a course correction, not a retreat— it's about being flexible and willing to adjust to achieve the best possible outcome.

3. **When to Pause**: Pausing is an often-overlooked but essential strategy for managing stress. When you feel overwhelmed, exhausted, or confused, it's important to take a step back and give yourself time to process. Pausing allows you to regain clarity, reduce emotional intensity, and make decisions with a calm and clear mind.

- ○ **Indicators to Pause**: Mental fatigue, emotional overwhelm, uncertainty about the next step. When you're in a state of high stress, pausing gives you the space to recalibrate, gather your thoughts, and approach the situation with fresh energy and focus.

## Conclusion:

Handling pressure like a pro is not about avoiding stress or trying to eliminate it entirely. It's about learning how to manage stress in a way that enhances your performance, decision-making, and emotional resilience. By using crisis management tactics from high-performing individuals, practicing tools like tactical breathing, box thinking, and decision anchors, and finding the balance between logic and emotion, you can navigate high-pressure situations with confidence and clarity.

The ability to know when to push, when to pivot, and when to pause is an essential skill for success in both your personal and professional life. Stress, when managed effectively, can become a driving force that propels you toward success, rather than a source of overwhelm. By cultivating these skills, you can turn pressure into progress and handle life's challenges with the poise and strength of a true high performer.

# Chapter 12

# Redefining Strength — The New Male Code

**Introduction:**

For generations, the idea of strength in men has been rooted in outward appearances: muscular bodies, dominance in social settings, the ability to 'take on the world,' and, in some cases, even the willingness to endure suffering for the sake of appearances. It's a model of masculinity that's defined by external validation, competitive prowess, and a narrow understanding of what it means to be truly strong. Yet, as society evolves and the pressures on men continue to shift, there is a growing awareness that the traditional concept of strength—while admirable in some respects—is ultimately incomplete.

In the 21st century, men are realizing that true strength is not always measured by how loudly they speak, how much they can lift, or how fiercely they assert themselves. True strength comes from within. It's about internal clarity, emotional intelligence, resilience, and the ability to show up in a way that feels authentic to who you are—without seeking constant validation from others. The new male code doesn't ask men to compete or dominate; it invites them to redefine their understanding of strength and embrace a more holistic, authentic version of masculinity.

This chapter will explore the evolution of masculinity and redefine what it means to be strong in today's world. We'll look at the shift from seeking external validation to cultivating internal clarity. We'll break down what strength looks like in a modern man and discuss how letting go of outdated myths—such as the "hero myth" that demands men to "die on every hill"—can free them from unnecessary burdens. Finally, we'll discuss how to integrate qualities like confidence, calm, and quiet power into your life, creating a version of strength that is as much about peace as it is about performance.

By the end of this chapter, you will have a clearer understanding of how to cultivate a more authentic and grounded form of strength—one that empowers you to live with clarity, confidence, and purpose.

## Shifting from External Validation to Internal Clarity

For most of history, men were taught to seek their worth from external sources—how much money they made, how they performed at work, how many people respected them, or how physically powerful they appeared. These markers of validation were external, visible, and often rooted in competition with others. The idea was that the more you dominated or succeeded in these areas, the stronger you would be perceived by society and, therefore, yourself.

However, this external validation comes at a high cost. When strength is defined by external metrics, men become reliant on the approval of others to feel good about themselves. They base their sense of self-worth on how they are perceived, how much praise they receive, and whether they are accepted by the social circles they inhabit. The result is a constant cycle of seeking validation, trying to measure up to others' standards, and feeling empty when that external recognition inevitably fades.

The shift from external validation to internal clarity is at the heart of redefining strength in modern men. Internal clarity is about understanding who you are, what you stand for, and what you want out of life—without needing constant affirmation from others. It's about recognizing that your worth is not determined by how many people admire you, but by how deeply you understand and accept yourself.

1. **Self-Awareness**: Internal clarity begins with self-awareness. It's about understanding your values, strengths, weaknesses, and desires. By taking the time to reflect on your life and identify what truly matters to you, you can begin to make decisions that align with your authentic self, rather than trying to live up to someone else's expectations.

2. **Self-Compassion**: Part of the journey to internal clarity is learning to treat yourself with kindness and understanding, especially when you fall short of your own expectations. Instead of punishing yourself for perceived failures, embrace the idea that mistakes are part of the process and allow yourself to grow from them.

3. **Letting Go of the Need for Approval**: Cultivating internal clarity means letting go of the constant need for approval from others. It's about accepting that you can't control what people think of you, and that their judgments do not define you. When

you no longer base your identity on the approval of others, you free yourself to live authentically and make choices based on your own beliefs and values.

4. **Living with Purpose**: Internal clarity also involves aligning your actions with a deeper sense of purpose. By identifying your true passions and long-term goals, you can begin to live with intention, moving through life with a sense of direction that doesn't depend on external feedback. Purpose becomes your anchor, guiding you through life's challenges and giving you the strength to endure even the toughest times.

As you make the shift from external validation to internal clarity, you begin to redefine what strength looks like. It's no longer about how others perceive you, but about how you perceive yourself—your ability to stand firm in your values and pursue your own truth.

## What Strength Looks Like in a Modern Man

In the past, strength was often defined in physical terms: the ability to fight, the capacity to provide, or the dominance in social situations. While these forms of strength are still valuable, they represent only a small fraction of what it means to be a strong man in the modern world.

True strength in the modern context is multifaceted—it goes beyond physical prowess and extends into emotional intelligence, mental fortitude, and the ability to navigate life's complexities with resilience and balance.

1. **Emotional Strength**: Emotional strength is often overlooked in traditional definitions of masculinity, but it is one of the most important forms of strength a man can cultivate. This includes the ability to recognize and regulate emotions, communicate effectively, and show empathy without losing control of one's own emotional well-being. An emotionally strong man is not afraid to express vulnerability, seek help when needed, or offer support to others in times of need.

2. **Mental Strength**: Mental strength is the ability to persevere in the face of adversity, stay focused on goals, and maintain resilience when challenges arise. It involves developing a growth mindset—understanding that setbacks are opportunities to learn and grow. Mentally strong men don't allow failure to define them; instead, they use it as fuel to push forward and continue their journey with renewed determination.

3. **Physical Strength**: While physical strength remains an important aspect of a man's health and well-being, it no longer defines his worth or value. Modern men understand that physical fitness is just one aspect of strength. It supports mental clarity, emotional stability, and overall well-being, but it's not the sole determinant of strength. A strong man takes care of his body, but he also prioritizes his emotional and mental health.

4. **Relational Strength**: Relationships are a cornerstone of a fulfilling life. A strong man builds and nurtures relationships based on trust, communication, and mutual respect. He is willing

to show up for his loved ones, listen deeply, and support them without trying to control or fix everything. Relational strength is rooted in empathy, kindness, and a willingness to invest in the people who matter most.

In a modern context, strength is not about dominating others or proving superiority—it's about creating balance, maintaining integrity, and building resilience in all areas of life. It's a quiet, steady strength that doesn't seek validation but instead grows from within.

## Letting Go of the Outdated Hero Myth (You Don't Need to Die on Every Hill)

For generations, men have been socialized to embody the "hero myth"—a narrative that champions self-sacrifice, relentless pursuit of success, and an unwavering commitment to protecting others, often at the expense of their own well-being. The hero is the one who "dies on every hill," who fights tirelessly and with no regard for the personal toll it takes.

While the hero myth has served as a powerful archetype throughout history, it's time to let go of this outdated notion of strength. The idea that men must sacrifice themselves on every hill they climb is both unrealistic and unsustainable. No one, especially men, should be expected to carry the weight of the world on their shoulders without seeking support, acknowledging their limitations, or prioritizing their own health and happiness.

Here's why it's time to let go of the hero myth:

1. **Sacrificing Yourself Doesn't Equal Strength**: The hero myth often equates self-sacrifice with strength, but this is a misconception. True strength lies in knowing when to stand your ground and when to step back. It's about being able to choose the battles that matter and not exhausting yourself on every trivial conflict that comes your way. A strong man knows that he doesn't need to prove himself by constantly sacrificing his time, energy, or well-being for others.

2. **Sustainability Over Burnout**: Men who constantly buy into the hero myth tend to burn out. They push themselves beyond their limits, believing that their worth is measured by how much they can endure. But this approach is unsustainable. Real strength involves maintaining balance—recognizing when you need to rest, recover, and recharge in order to be effective in the long term. Burnout isn't a badge of honor—it's a sign that something needs to change.

3. **Letting Go of Perfectionism**: The hero myth encourages perfectionism, making men feel that they must always succeed, always excel, and always do more. But no one can be perfect, and no one can succeed all the time. Strength is about resilience, not perfection. It's about learning to adapt, evolve, and grow, even when things don't go as planned.

4. **Embracing Collaboration, Not Lone Wolf Mentality**: The hero myth often portrays men as lone wolves—individuals who take on the world alone and reject help from others. However,

the strength of modern masculinity is rooted in collaboration and community. Strong men are not afraid to ask for help, lean on others, or work as part of a team. True strength comes from knowing when to rely on others and recognizing that you don't have to do everything alone.

## Integrating Confidence, Calm, and Quiet Power

True strength in modern men is not about dominating the room or raising your voice to assert yourself—it's about embodying quiet power, confidence, and calm under pressure. This form of strength doesn't seek to control or overpower others, but instead radiates an inner assurance that commands respect without needing to be loud or aggressive.

1. **Confidence Without Arrogance**: Confidence is the belief in your abilities and worth, but it doesn't require arrogance or superiority. Confident men understand their strengths and limitations, and they are comfortable in their own skin. They don't need to prove themselves to others because they have already proven their value to themselves. Confidence comes from a deep internal foundation, not from seeking external approval.

2. **Calm in the Chaos**: One of the most powerful aspects of modern strength is the ability to stay calm under pressure. The world is chaotic, and challenges are inevitable. But men who are able to remain calm in the midst of turmoil are able to think more clearly, make better decisions, and lead with grace. Calmness is a form of emotional intelligence—it allows you to manage your responses and navigate stressful situations with clarity.

3. **Quiet Power**: Quiet power is the ability to influence and lead without force or aggression. It's the power of self-awareness, emotional regulation, and purposeful action. Quietly powerful men know that their value doesn't need to be shouted from the rooftops—they lead by example, and their actions speak louder than their words. This type of power doesn't seek attention or validation; it simply exists as a result of consistent integrity and authenticity.

## Conclusion:

Redefining strength in the modern man means moving away from outdated stereotypes of heroism and embracing a more holistic, authentic version of masculinity. True strength lies in internal clarity, emotional intelligence, and the ability to maintain balance in all areas of life. It's about confidence without arrogance, calmness under pressure, and quiet power that commands respect without needing to assert dominance.

By letting go of the need for external validation, embracing vulnerability, and focusing on what truly matters, men can cultivate a new type of strength—one that is grounded in authenticity, emotional resilience, and purposeful action. This new male code encourages men to lead with integrity, support each other, and redefine what it means to be strong in today's complex world.

# Chapter 13

# The No-Therapy Game Plan — A Framework for Self-Mastery

## Introduction:

The world often tells men that emotional health requires professional help—therapy, counseling, and guided sessions that lead you through the layers of your psyche. While therapy can undoubtedly be beneficial for many, there's a growing understanding that self-mastery doesn't always have to come with a therapist's chair or a counselor's office. Men, particularly in a world that's always moving forward and focused on achievement, need a system they can rely on to manage their mental and emotional health without feeling dependent on external support. A self-check system—a framework for managing your own well-being—is more than possible; it's necessary.

In this chapter, we'll dive into how you can build your own mental health framework—an internal game plan that allows you to assess and improve your emotional health without needing therapy as the crutch. This system will be uniquely yours, based on your values, your daily wins, your discipline, and your ability to reflect on where you are and where you want to go. Most importantly, it will offer accountability without shame, and will teach you how to navigate challenges and grow without being paralyzed by your weaknesses.

By the end of this chapter, you will understand how to build a self-sustaining mental health system that supports your journey of self-mastery and personal growth. It's time to take control, create your own "code," and build a life that reflects the true strength and resilience you're capable of.

## How to Build a Self-Check System for Mental Health Without Therapy

Building a self-check system for your mental health isn't about ignoring the importance of external support—it's about creating a sustainable practice of self-awareness and self-regulation that empowers you to manage stress, emotions, and life's challenges independently. By developing a structured way to monitor and assess your emotional state, you can prevent burnout, emotional overload, and mental fatigue before they become overwhelming.

1. **Daily Self-Assessment**: One of the simplest ways to maintain mental health is through regular self-assessment. This involves taking a few minutes each day to reflect on how you're feeling emotionally and mentally. You can do this through a quick self-inventory:

   o **What did I feel today?** Did I feel stressed, happy, frustrated, or calm?

   o **How did I react to challenges?** Was I able to manage my emotions, or did I overreact?

○ **What did I accomplish today?** Reflect on the wins and the things you did well, no matter how small.

○ **What do I need to address?** Is there something emotionally significant that you're avoiding or haven't processed?

This practice of self-checking helps you stay aware of your mental health and gives you the ability to identify patterns, triggers, or issues that might need attention. By assessing yourself daily, you can make minor course corrections in real time, rather than allowing your emotional state to spiral unchecked.

2. **Weekly Reflection**: While daily self-checks help you monitor your mental health on a micro level, a weekly reflection allows you to zoom out and look at the bigger picture. Take time each week to evaluate your progress, review your goals, and assess how you handled challenges over the past few days.

○ **What were the highlights of the week?** Identify what went well, and how you performed.

○ **Where did I struggle?** Reflect on areas where you may have fallen short, emotionally or mentally, and why that might have happened.

○ **How did I manage stress and frustration?** Did you fall into any negative patterns? If so, what caused it, and how can you do better next week?

- ○ **What could I improve next week?** Identify concrete actions you can take to improve your mental well-being, whether it's setting aside time for self-care, improving sleep, or tackling a challenging emotional issue.

By reviewing your week, you gain a broader perspective on your mental and emotional health, allowing you to celebrate successes and adjust behaviors where necessary. This reflection helps you learn from experience and stay on track with your personal growth.

3. **Monthly Check-In**: Every month, conduct a more thorough review of your mental health and progress. Ask yourself larger, more reflective questions like:

  - ○ **Have I been consistent in managing stress?** Reflect on whether your daily practices and routines have supported your mental well-being.

  - ○ **What habits do I need to break or start?** This is an opportunity to evaluate whether certain behaviors or habits are negatively impacting your mental health, and to decide on actionable steps to change them.

  - ○ **Am I meeting my emotional needs?** Emotional health requires self-compassion and the ability to understand and meet your needs. Ask yourself whether you've been taking the time to nurture your emotional health, build connections, and practice self-care.

The monthly check-in allows you to take a more comprehensive view of your mental state. It's a chance to reset and adjust your approach to life, ensuring that you're on the right track toward long-term mental health and self-mastery.

## Create Your "Code": Values, Daily Wins, Discipline, Reflection

At the core of any self-mastery plan is a personal code—your own set of values, principles, and practices that guide your decisions and behavior. Building your "code" is about defining what truly matters to you, how you want to live, and the habits and behaviors that support that vision.

1.  **Define Your Values**: Values are the foundation of your mental health and personal growth. They represent what is most important to you, and they guide every decision and action you take. Some common values might include integrity, respect, family, health, or personal growth.

    o   **How to Define Your Values**: To define your values, think about moments in your life when you felt most fulfilled or proud. What were you doing in those moments? What did you stand for? What principles were guiding you? Write down the values that resonate with you most deeply, and consider how you can embody them in your daily life.

2. **Track Your Daily Wins**: Building a "win" mentality is key to sustaining motivation and building momentum. Every day, find something to celebrate, even if it's small. Acknowledging your achievements, whether it's completing a challenging task at work, maintaining focus during a tough conversation, or sticking to your fitness goals, helps build confidence and reinforces a positive mental state.

   ○ **How to Track Your Wins**: Each day, write down at least one thing you accomplished, regardless of how small it may seem. This helps you maintain focus on progress rather than dwelling on setbacks or failures. Over time, you'll notice a pattern of success that boosts your confidence and sense of purpose.

3. **Discipline as Freedom**: Discipline is often misunderstood as restrictive, but it's actually liberating. Having the discipline to create and maintain healthy habits gives you the freedom to perform at your best, stay grounded, and manage stress more effectively. When you create a routine that supports your mental health, your emotional resilience improves, and you begin to feel more in control of your life.

   ○ **Building Discipline**: Discipline is built through small, consistent actions. Whether it's making your bed every morning, sticking to a workout routine, or planning your day the night before, discipline starts with the small things. Over time, these actions become habits, and those habits create the structure that supports your mental well-being.

4. **Daily Reflection**: As mentioned earlier, daily reflection is a key part of your self-check system. It involves looking at your actions, emotions, and decisions each day and making necessary adjustments. Through reflection, you can assess whether your actions are in alignment with your values and whether you're staying on track toward your goals.

   o **How to Reflect**: Every evening, take a few minutes to reflect on your day. Ask yourself:

     ■ What went well today?

     ■ Where did I fall short?

     ■ How did I handle stress, frustration, and other emotions?

     ■ What can I do better tomorrow?

By incorporating daily reflection into your routine, you create an opportunity to fine-tune your approach to life and make continuous improvements to your mental health and emotional well-being.

## Accountability Without Shame

One of the most powerful aspects of self-mastery is accountability. But accountability doesn't have to involve external pressure or shame. True accountability is about taking responsibility for your actions and making a commitment to yourself to show up every day.

116

1. **Self-Accountability**: Self-accountability means holding yourself responsible for your actions, your progress, and your well-being. It's about making commitments to yourself and following through, even when no one is watching. This internal accountability builds integrity and strengthens your self-esteem.

   o **How to Practice Self-Accountability**: Set clear goals for yourself—both short-term and long-term—and check in regularly to see how you're progressing. Instead of waiting for external validation, make it a point to acknowledge your own efforts and adjust your approach when needed. Celebrate your wins and hold yourself to a higher standard.

2. **Supportive Accountability**: While self-accountability is important, it can also be helpful to have a support system that holds you accountable without judgment. This might include a close friend, mentor, or group of like-minded individuals who can offer encouragement, provide feedback, and help you stay on track with your goals.

   o **How to Create Supportive Accountability**: Find someone who aligns with your values and who is invested in your growth. This could be a trusted friend, a workout buddy, or a mentor who can check in on your progress and offer guidance. The key is to create a relationship built on trust and mutual support, not on shame or guilt.

## The Roadmap to Becoming Hardwired and Human— On Your Terms

The ultimate goal of creating your own game plan for mental health and self-mastery is to live life on your terms. This means having the mental clarity and emotional resilience to navigate life's challenges without losing your sense of self. You become "hardwired" in the sense that you've built a system of habits, values, and practices that support your well-being. But you also remain "human" in the sense that you accept imperfection, embrace vulnerability, and prioritize growth over perfection.

To build a life that's "hardwired and human," consider the following:

1. **Define Your Own Success**: Your roadmap to self-mastery begins with defining what success looks like for you. Don't let society's standards dictate your sense of accomplishment. Focus on what truly matters—whether it's building meaningful relationships, pursuing personal passions, or achieving professional goals. When you define your own success, you set yourself up for a life that's aligned with your values.

2. **Embrace Imperfection**: Perfection is an illusion. Rather than striving for flawless execution, embrace the process of growth. Mistakes are opportunities to learn, and setbacks are chances to build resilience. By accepting imperfection, you free yourself from the pressure to "get it right" all the time.

3. **Live Authentically**: Your game plan for self-mastery should be aligned with who you truly are. Don't try to fit into someone

else's mold—create a life that reflects your true values, desires, and aspirations. When you live authentically, you build strength from within and develop the clarity to navigate life's challenges with confidence.

## Conclusion:

Building a self-check system for mental health and self-mastery is not about perfection or relying on external validation. It's about creating a personalized framework that allows you to stay grounded, focused, and resilient in the face of life's challenges. By developing your "code"—your values, daily wins, discipline, and reflections—you create a system that supports your mental well-being and helps you achieve your goals on your terms.

With accountability, self-reflection, and a commitment to living authentically, you can become the best version of yourself, hardwired for success while staying connected to your humanity. Through consistent effort, self-awareness, and growth, you can create a life of purpose and strength, and master your mental health without needing therapy as a crutch. The power is in your hands—it's time to take control and live life on your terms.

# A Message to Men Who Feel Seen for the First Time

As you reach the end of this journey through the evolution of modern masculinity, there's something you must know: You are not alone.

For too long, many men have felt isolated in their struggles. Whether it's the weight of societal expectations, the constant pressure to be "tough" or "successful," or the sense of emotional disconnect that comes from bottling things up, men often carry a silent burden that goes unspoken. This feeling of isolation—the sense that no one understands or even acknowledges the complexity of what it means to be a man today—can be suffocating. But here's the truth: you're not alone. You've simply been conditioned not to speak up.

For generations, men were taught to keep their emotions in check, to be self-reliant to the point of silence, and to measure their worth in terms of what they could achieve. But things are changing. More men are embracing the idea that vulnerability, authenticity, and emotional intelligence are not weaknesses—they are strengths. And if this book has made you feel seen for the first time, know that you are part of a larger movement. A movement of men who are finally stepping out of the shadows, who are redefining what it means to be truly strong, who are allowing themselves to live real lives—lives that are as grounded in emotional clarity as they are in action and achievement.

The emotional labyrinth that you've been navigating doesn't have to be a solo journey. Many men have walked this path before you and many more will walk beside you. It's not about pretending to be something you're not or burying your pain—it's about being strong enough to admit that you need to evolve. The good news is, as you embrace this evolution, you'll find that the world isn't as lonely as it might seem. The more honest you are with yourself, the more you will find others who are walking the same path, ready to walk with you, side by side.

This epilogue is a reminder to you that being human doesn't mean being weak; it means being willing to embrace the full spectrum of who you are, and to lean into the strength that vulnerability offers. And in doing so, you will discover the quiet courage that lies within, the courage to live authentically, without the need to fit into outdated molds.

## Resources, Routines, and Books/Tools for Solo Growth

While the journey of self-mastery and emotional clarity is an ongoing one, there are countless resources to help you grow and develop into the man you want to become. You don't have to do this alone. There are tools, routines, and practices that can guide you through the process of integrating your emotional health, mental clarity, and physical well-being.

Here are some resources, books, and routines that can support your solo growth:

1. **Books**:

- *The Power of Now* by Eckhart Tolle: A transformative book that teaches you the importance of living in the present moment, focusing on the here and now rather than constantly worrying about the past or future.

- *Man's Search for Meaning* by Viktor E. Frankl: Frankl's reflections on surviving the Holocaust and his psychological insights into finding meaning in life are powerful lessons on resilience and purpose.

- *The Art of Manliness* by Brett McKay: This book combines timeless wisdom with practical advice on living a purposeful and intentional life as a modern man.

- *Dare to Lead* by Brené Brown: Brown's work on vulnerability, courage, and leadership is invaluable for men who wish to cultivate emotional intelligence and resilience without sacrificing their masculinity.

2. **Tools**:

- **Journaling**: Whether it's free-flow journaling, bullet points, or guided prompts, journaling can help you process your emotions and clarify your thoughts. You don't need to do it every day, but integrating it into your routine helps in maintaining emotional clarity.

- **Meditation & Mindfulness Apps**: Apps like Headspace, Calm, or Insight Timer can provide short guided meditations that help you stay grounded and

122

reduce stress. Mindfulness isn't just a trendy buzzword; it's a powerful tool for self-awareness and emotional regulation.

o **Daily Habits Tracker**: Using a habits tracker can be an excellent way to stay on track with your goals. You can track physical health, mental health, and other self-improvement goals. The visual reminder of progress builds momentum.

3. **Routines**:

o **Morning Routine**: Start your day with intention. This could include meditation, journaling, exercise, or even reading. Having a morning routine helps you focus your energy and set a positive tone for the day.

o **Evening Reflection**: Take time in the evening to reflect on the day's wins and challenges. Ask yourself what you did well, what could be improved, and what you're grateful for. This habit ensures you close the day with clarity and sets the foundation for a good night's sleep.

o **Physical Activity**: Regular exercise is not only good for the body but also the mind. It helps to release stress, improve mood, and increase mental clarity. Whether it's lifting weights, going for a run, or practicing yoga, find what works for you and make it a part of your routine.

4. **Therapeutic Alternatives**:

   ○ **Talk to a Friend**: If you don't feel ready for therapy but want to speak about your emotions, try confiding in a trusted friend or mentor. Having someone to listen, without judgment, can help you process your thoughts and feelings.

   ○ **Creative Expression**: Sometimes, it's not about talking; it's about expressing. Whether through music, art, writing, or another form of creative expression, these outlets can help you process and release emotions that words sometimes cannot.

   ○ **Nature Walks**: Stepping outside and being in nature can have profound mental health benefits. A walk through the park, a hike in the mountains, or simply sitting in nature can help clear your mind and give you a fresh perspective on your challenges.

## Quiet Courage: The Power of Living Real, Not Just Tough

As men, we are often told that strength means being tough—that strength is about physical endurance, stoicism, and always standing tall, no matter the cost. But in today's world, the greatest strength doesn't come from forcing your way through life. It comes from having the courage to live authentically, to embrace both your strengths and vulnerabilities, and to pursue a life that reflects your true self.

The quiet courage of living real is about:

1. **Embracing Vulnerability**: Real strength doesn't come from hiding your emotions or pretending to be invincible. It comes from embracing vulnerability—the courage to show up as yourself, to admit when you don't have all the answers, and to ask for help when you need it. This takes far more strength than simply putting on a brave face.

2. **Practicing Self-Compassion**: Strength isn't about being hard on yourself or pushing through pain. It's about being kind to yourself, forgiving your mistakes, and understanding that growth is a process. Self-compassion allows you to heal, grow, and improve without being weighed down by self-criticism.

3. **Leading by Example**: The quietest form of strength is the ability to lead by example—not through grand gestures or flashy displays of power, but through everyday actions. When you live with integrity, when you treat others with respect, when you show up consistently and thoughtfully, you demonstrate the kind of strength that inspires those around you without saying a word.

4. **Building Emotional Resilience**: Life will continue to present challenges. The power lies not in avoiding the storms, but in learning how to face them with emotional resilience. Resilience isn't about never being shaken; it's about bouncing back, learning from your experiences, and continuing forward despite setbacks.

Living real—living in alignment with your true self, your values, and your beliefs—is the ultimate act of strength. It is the strength that allows you to be flexible, adaptive, and deeply connected to who you are. It's about accepting that while life may challenge you, you are capable of handling it on your own terms.

## Conclusion:

As you step away from this book, I want you to know that you are not alone in your journey. The world may sometimes feel like it's asking you to be someone you're not, but true strength lies in the ability to walk through life as your authentic self—grounded, resilient, and unshaken by the expectations of others.

Your journey toward self-mastery, emotional resilience, and authentic living isn't about perfection—it's about progress. It's about continuing to build yourself, one step at a time, with a focus on values, integrity, and emotional clarity. You don't need therapy to figure it all out, but you do need to develop your own framework for growth and self-understanding. The tools and practices outlined in this book are meant to empower you to walk that path with confidence and courage.

In the quiet courage of living real—of embracing your vulnerabilities, confronting your challenges, and living on your own terms—you will discover the most powerful form of strength: a strength that is grounded in your humanity. And that strength will serve you for a lifetime, through all the highs and lows that come with being truly human. You are enough, just as you are.

# Epilogue

## The Journey to True Strength and Self-Mastery

As we close this journey through the evolving landscape of modern masculinity, it's clear that the path to strength and self-mastery is not defined by the traditional ideals we have inherited from the past. The message from these 13 chapters is simple, yet profound: True strength is not found in external validation, relentless sacrifice, or rigid stereotypes of what it means to be a man. Instead, real strength lies in the quiet power of self-awareness, emotional intelligence, and the ability to live authentically and intentionally.

In the first few chapters, we explored how men have been conditioned to wear masks—strength, resilience, and stoicism—often at the cost of emotional well-being. We discussed the silent epidemic of emotional distress, where high-functioning men, despite outward success, struggle with inner turmoil. But the strength to break free from this cycle lies not in further suppressing our emotions but in learning how to process them, step by step. As we've seen, men can redefine their strength by breaking the outdated hero myth and choosing to focus on emotional resilience, empathy, and self-care.

Moving through the chapters, we learned that strength comes from within. It starts with shifting from external validation to internal clarity. This isn't just a theoretical concept; it's a practical shift toward understanding who you are, what you value, and how you want to show up in the world. When you begin to trust yourself, make decisions aligned with your values, and stop seeking constant approval, you unlock an authentic version of strength. Internal clarity is the compass that guides you when life becomes chaotic.

Throughout these pages, we emphasized that real power is not about dominance or control—it's about balance. In redefining strength, we explored how to integrate confidence, calm, and quiet power into our lives. The ability to remain calm under pressure, make decisions with clarity, and act with confidence comes from a deep understanding of oneself. The quiet strength is one that doesn't seek to prove anything to others but instead lives with intention, staying grounded and aligned with one's core values.

This journey also delved into practical tools for handling stress, emotional overload, and mental health. Building a self-check system for mental health without the need for therapy was a central theme. We discussed how to develop a system of daily self-assessment, weekly reflection, and monthly check-ins to keep your mental state in check, empowering you to take control of your emotional health. Building a "code"—a personal set of values, routines, and habits—helps you navigate life with purpose and direction, ensuring that you are not at the mercy of external pressures or fleeting emotions.

Perhaps the most empowering takeaway from this journey is that you do not need to do this alone. While the path to self-mastery is personal, it does not have to be solitary. Whether through accountability partners, trusted friends, or communities of like-minded men, support is crucial in sustaining progress. True strength is found in shared humanity, in the willingness to lean on others and to offer support in return.

In the end, this book is about reclaiming your humanity in the face of external pressures, societal expectations, and internal doubts. It's about recognizing that your strength is defined by your ability to be authentic, resilient, and emotionally intelligent—not by how well you fit into the outdated molds of manhood that no longer serve you. The roadmap provided in these chapters is a guide to help you move from a place of confusion, frustration, or disconnection to a life of purpose, peace, and power.

By redefining what it means to be a man and focusing on emotional and mental clarity, confidence, and strength, you can lead a life that is deeply aligned with who you truly are. You are capable of becoming a man who embodies quiet courage—the courage to live real, not just tough. This is your journey, and it's time to step into your full potential with a clear mind, a strong heart, and the unshakable power of self-mastery.

www.ingramcontent.com/pod-product-compliance
Lightning Source LLC
Chambersburg PA
CBHW070120030426
42335CB00016B/2218